AF268753

Pelvic Floor Exercises for Senior Women Over 60

A 4-Week Illustrated Workout Guide to Build Core Strength, Regain
Bladder Control, and Move Freely with Confidence

Calla Holt

Copyright © 2026 by Calla Holt

All rights reserved. No part of this publication may be reproduced, distributed, or transmitted in any form or by any means, including photocopying, recording, or other electronic or mechanical methods, without the prior written permission of the author, except in the case of brief quotations embodied in critical reviews and certain other noncommercial uses permitted by copyright law.

Disclaimer

This book is intended for general informational and educational purposes only. The exercises and guidance contained in this publication are not a substitute for professional medical advice, diagnosis, or treatment. Always consult your physician or qualified healthcare provider before beginning any new exercise program, particularly if you have a pre-existing medical condition, recent injury, or surgery.

The author and publisher assume no responsibility for any injury, loss, or damage incurred as a result of the use or application of information contained in this book.

Dedication

This book is for the woman who has spent years becoming an expert at managing symptoms she was never properly taught to address.

For the one who quietly reorganized her schedule, her wardrobe, her choices, and her confidence around a problem nobody talked about openly. Who kept going. Who kept showing up. Who never stopped moving, even when moving felt uncertain.

For the woman who picked up this book because she decided that understanding her own body is not a luxury. It is something she is owed.

And for every woman at the beginning of that decision. The one who is not sure yet whether anything can change. The one who is giving it one more try.

This is for her too. Especially her.

You were right to keep looking.

Contents

Introduction

It happened at a dinner party. You were laughing, properly laughing, the kind that catches you off guard and takes over before you can prepare for it. And in the middle of that laughter, you felt it. A small, unwelcome dampness. You shifted in your chair, kept smiling, and spent the next hour calculating whether it was noticeable. You left earlier than you had planned.

If that moment sounds familiar, or some version of it does, you are exactly in the right place. Not because pelvic floor problems are something you simply have to live with. But because they are something you can actually do something about, at any age, at any fitness level, starting right now.

I have worked with women on pelvic floor health and core rehabilitation for over twenty years. I have sat across from women in their sixties, seventies, and eighties who had quietly reorganized their entire lives around a bathroom. Women who stopped walking long distances, declined holidays, gave up exercise classes they loved, all without ever telling anyone why. The conversations I have had in those rooms are the reason this book exists.

This is not a medical treatment. It is a movement guide built on the same principles I use with women in my practice: correct breathing, coordinated muscle training, and a structured progressive program that fits into a real life. It works because it addresses the whole system, not just one part of it. You do not need a gym, equipment, or a background in fitness. You need this book and about fifteen to twenty minutes a day.

What This Book Gives You

There are four things this program is designed to deliver. The first is core strength: not the six-pack kind, but the deep internal support that keeps you upright, stable, and comfortable during everyday movement. The second is improved bladder control: fewer urgent dashes, less leakage, more confidence in the moments that matter. The third is freedom of movement: the ability to walk, bend, lift, and carry without bracing against your own body. The fourth is the quiet confidence that comes from knowing you have addressed the problem rather than worked around it.

How to Use This Book

Start with Part One. Chapters 1 and 2 give you the understanding you need to make the exercise work. Many women skip straight to the exercises and wonder why the results are inconsistent. The knowledge behind the movement matters. It takes less than an hour to read both chapters, and it will change how you approach everything that follows.

Part Two, Chapters 3 and 4, covers breathing, posture, and warm-up work. These are not optional extras. They are the foundation that makes the exercises in Parts Three and Four significantly more effective.

Part Three is the illustrated exercise library, organized by function: foundation exercises, core strength, bladder control, and mobility. You will use these chapters as reference material throughout the program and beyond.

Part Four contains the 4-week program in Chapter 9 and the long-term lifestyle guidance in Chapter 10. Begin the program only after reading Parts One and Two. The sequence is designed deliberately.

Your Starting Point Self-Assessment

Before you begin, take five minutes to complete this checklist honestly. Mark each item yes or no. Keep this page. You will return to it at the end of Week 4 and answer the same questions again. The comparison will tell you more than any scale or fitness test.

Self-Assessment: Your Starting Point

Answer yes or no to each question. This is for your eyes only.

☐ Do you leak urine when you sneeze, cough, laugh, or exercise, even a small amount?

□ Do you feel a sudden strong urge to reach the bathroom quickly, sometimes with little warning?

□ Do you visit the bathroom more than eight times during the day or more than once during the night?

□ Do you feel heaviness or pressure in your pelvic area, particularly after standing for a while?

□ Do you sometimes feel you cannot fully empty your bladder or bowel?

□ Do you experience lower back discomfort that worsens with activity or prolonged sitting?

□ Do you plan your outings around bathroom access or avoid certain activities because of bladder concerns?

□ Have you noticed changes in your posture or the way you move that you cannot fully explain?

Set that checklist aside. Do not try to fix everything before you begin. This is simply your starting point, and knowing it clearly is the most useful thing you can do right now.

The work starts on the next page. You are not behind. You are right on time.

Part I: Know Your Body

Chapter 1

Your Pelvic Floor at 60 and Beyond

These muscles have been working for you your entire life. They held things in place through pregnancies and long car journeys and decades of movement. They coordinated with your breathing without ever asking for your attention. And most women, until something shifts, have no real picture of what they are, where they sit, or what happens when they stop working at full capacity.

What It Is and What It Supports

Think of the underside of a suspension bridge. The roadway above carries traffic and weight, and the entire structure depends on what hangs below it: a network of cables and supports, taut and coordinated, holding everything in alignment under load. Your pelvic floor works in something like that way. It is not a single muscle but a layered group of muscles and connective tissues that stretch across the base of your pelvis, from your pubic bone at the front to your tailbone at the back, and from one sitting bone across to the other.

Those muscles are doing several jobs simultaneously. They hold your bladder, uterus, and bowel in their correct positions within the pelvis, preventing them from dropping downward under the constant force of gravity. They control the sphincter muscles that allow you to stay continent, opening and closing the urethra and rectum with coordination and intention. They work alongside your deep abdominal muscles and lower back to form part of the core support system that stabilizes your spine and pelvis every time you move, lift, or change position.

Because these muscles sit internally and do their work without any visible sign of effort, most women do not think about them until something changes. The first indication that something has shifted is usually functional: a cough that causes a leak, an urgency that arrives without much warning, a heaviness at the end of a long day. These are not signs that something has broken. They are signs that a muscle group that has been working hard for decades without any focused attention has finally started to show the wear.

What the pelvic floor supports extends beyond the obvious. Bladder and bowel control are the most commonly discussed functions, but the pelvic floor also plays a significant role in spinal stability. When the deep core system is working well, the diaphragm, the transverse abdominis, the lower back stabilizers, and the pelvic floor all activate together as a coordinated pressure management unit. A weakened or dysfunctional pelvic floor changes how the entire system works and how your back, hips, and posture respond to everyday demands.

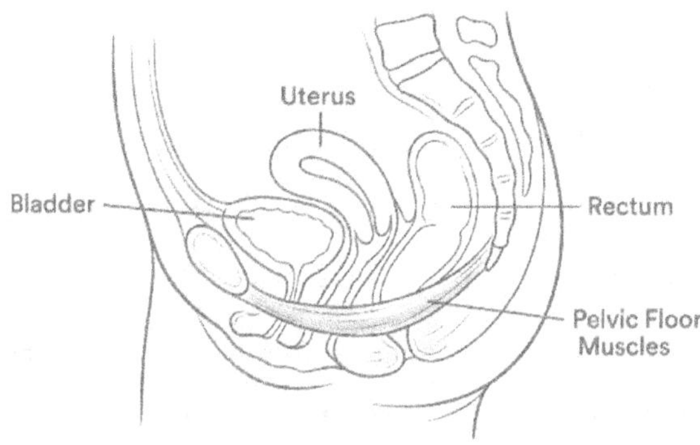

It also contributes to sexual sensation and function, something women are often not told directly but which matters to quality of life. Changes in sensation or comfort are not inevitable with age, and pelvic floor training can make a genuine difference in this area for many women.

Why It Weakens with Age and Hormonal Change

The pelvic floor does not weaken overnight. It happens gradually, across years, and through a combination of factors that are entirely normal and entirely addressable.

Estrogen is the central player. This hormone maintains the tone, elasticity, and thickness of pelvic floor muscles and the surrounding connective tissues and mucous membranes throughout your reproductive years. It keeps the tissue supple and the muscles responsive. After menopause, when estrogen production drops significantly, the muscles and tissues that depended on it begin to change. They become thinner, less elastic, and more prone to fatigue under load. The urethral lining, which estrogen also maintains, becomes drier and less cushioned, which can increase bladder sensitivity and cause a sudden urgency that was not there before.

Age itself contributes, independent of hormonal change. Like any muscle group that has not been consistently and specifically trained, the pelvic floor loses some of its coordination and fast-twitch response over time. The muscles that once reacted quickly and automatically to a cough or a sneeze begin to lag slightly behind the pressure spike. That lag is often where leakage happens.

For women who have had children, pregnancy and delivery added their own demands on these muscles decades ago. The stretching and potential tearing or trauma of childbirth can leave lasting effects on muscle coordination and strength that may not become noticeable until the additional factor of hormonal change arrives in midlife. A woman who managed perfectly well through her forties may find that symptoms she had quietly managed now become more significant in her sixties. That combination of old injury and new hormonal context is a common pattern, and it responds well to targeted training.

Lifestyle factors over the decades also leave their mark. Years of prolonged sitting, particularly in a rounded-forward posture, places constant downward pressure on the pelvic floor. High-impact activity without appropriate pelvic floor engagement can stress the muscles repeatedly. Even habitual breath-holding during exertion, something many women do without realizing it, creates repetitive pressure spikes that the pelvic floor absorbs without support from the rest of the core system. None of these factors cause irreversible damage. They simply explain why the muscles are starting from a different baseline than they once had.

Weak Floor Vs Tight Floor

This is the section that most pelvic floor books skip entirely, and it is one of the most important things you can understand before you begin any program.

A pelvic floor can present two very different kinds of dysfunction. The first is weakness: the muscles lack the strength, endurance, or coordination to do their job. The second is tension: the muscles are held in a state of chronic contraction and cannot release fully, which makes them unable to work through their proper range of motion. The frustrating thing about these two patterns is that they can produce symptoms that look almost identical from the outside: leakage, urgency, pelvic pressure, lower back discomfort.

A weak floor tends to present with stress leakage, meaning leakage that happens during physical exertion, coughing, sneezing, or laughing. There is a general sense that the muscles are not responding quickly enough or strongly enough to pressure events. Kegels, performed correctly, are an appropriate and effective response to this pattern. They build the strength and coordination the muscles need to hold under load.

A tight or overactive floor is a different picture. Women with this pattern often experience urgency, the sudden strong need to reach the bathroom, difficulty fully emptying the bladder or bowel, and sometimes a persistent sense of pressure or discomfort in the pelvic region. The muscles are not weak; they are chronically contracted and cannot lengthen properly. For this pattern, Kegels can make things considerably worse, because you are adding more contraction to muscles that are already over-contracted and desperately need to learn how to let go.

How do you get a general sense of which pattern might apply to you? A weak floor tends to involve leakage during activity, a feeling of reduced response or control, and symptoms that are worse toward the end of the day when the muscles are fatigued. A tight floor more often involves urgency rather than effort-related leakage, difficulty with complete emptying, and symptoms that can be worse after periods of stress or inactivity, when the muscles have been held in tension without release.

Many women have elements of both patterns, with some areas of the pelvic floor underactive and others holding excessive tension. This is why the program in this book addresses both directions of pelvic floor function: the strengthening work for the weak floor and the release and coordination work for the tight one. Chapter 5 introduces the Reverse Kegel alongside the Basic Kegel for exactly this reason. If you suspect you may have a predominantly tight floor, a session with a pelvic floor physiotherapist can give you a precise assessment and confirm which exercises to prioritize.

A Note on Self-Assessment

Reading these descriptions can help you begin to understand your own pattern, but it is not a diagnosis. Pelvic floor dysfunction exists on a spectrum, and the same symptom can have different causes in different women. Use the information here to build awareness and to approach the exercises with the right intention. If your symptoms are significant or have not responded to self-directed exercise before, the guidance in Chapter 10 on when to seek professional support is worth reading before you begin.

Signs Your Pelvic Floor Needs Attention Now

The following ten signs are all common among women over 60. None of them are unusual. None of them are permanent. Read through them and note which ones apply to you. This is not a list designed to make you feel worse about where you are starting. It is a map of what the program ahead is designed to address.

1. **Leaking when you sneeze, cough, laugh, or exercise.** Even a small amount counts. This is the most recognizable form of pelvic floor weakness and one of the most directly responsive to the exercises in this program.

2. **A sudden strong urge to reach the bathroom quickly.** Sometimes arriving with little warning and sometimes accompanied by leakage before you get there. This pattern is addressed specifically in Chapter 7.

3. **Needing the bathroom more than eight times during the day.** Or waking more than once at night when your fluid intake does not seem to explain it. Frequency without a clear cause is often a sign of a bladder that has become overly sensitive.

4. **A sense of heaviness or pressure in the pelvic area.** Particularly after standing for a period or at the end of a busy day. This can be associated with pelvic organ support changes and is worth mentioning to your doctor if it is persistent.

5. Difficulty fully emptying your bladder or bowel. The feeling that something remains even after you have finished. This can be connected to a tight or poorly coordinating pelvic floor that does not release fully during the process of elimination.

6. Lower back ache that worsens after activity or prolonged sitting. The pelvic floor and lower back muscles work as part of the same core stability system. When one is underperforming, the other tends to compensate and fatigue more quickly.

7. A change in posture you have noticed in yourself. A tendency to lean forward slightly, shift your weight, shorten your stride, or move more carefully than you used to without a specific injury to explain it.

8. Reduced confidence in physical activity. Avoiding exercise classes, long walks, or social situations that involve physical activity because of uncertainty about bladder control. The social and emotional effect of pelvic floor symptoms is real and rarely discussed.

9. Discomfort or changed sensation in the pelvic region. Not acute pain, but a persistent awareness, dryness, or discomfort that was not there before. Often connected to the tissue changes that accompany the drop in estrogen after menopause.

10. The quiet daily workarounds you have built without naming them. Knowing the location of every bathroom before you arrive somewhere new. Wearing dark clothing as a precaution. Reducing how much you drink before leaving the house. Sitting toward the aisle in a theatre. These adjustments are so normalized they may not feel like symptoms anymore. They are.

Every item on this list is something I hear regularly from women who have come to me having managed these issues quietly for months or years. Every one of them is something the program in this book directly addresses. Not all at once, and not all equally quickly, but genuinely and progressively over the four weeks ahead. The starting point is understanding what is happening and why. You now have that. The next chapter gives you the one piece that most books about pelvic floor health leave out entirely.

Chapter 2

The Missing Link Most Books Skip

Pick up almost any pelvic floor book and you will find the same instruction on page one: do your Kegels. Squeeze, hold, release. Repeat. It is not wrong advice. But for many women, it is incomplete advice, and incomplete is often the reason a Kegel routine that starts with real commitment quietly fades after six weeks with little to show for it.

This chapter explains what is missing and why it matters. Once you understand how the pelvic floor connects to the rest of your core system, the exercises in this book will make more sense, and the results will come faster and last longer.

Why Kegels Alone Are Not Always Enough

A Kegel is a voluntary contraction of the pelvic floor muscles. Done correctly and consistently, it builds strength and coordination in the muscles responsible for bladder control and pelvic organ support. For women whose pelvic floor is genuinely weak and underactive, Kegels are an effective starting point. The muscles respond to the load, coordination improves, and over time, control gets better.

The problem begins when Kegels are the only tool in the box. The pelvic floor does not work in isolation. It functions as part of a four-muscle pressure system that includes your diaphragm, your deep abdominal muscles, and your lower back stabilizers. When you perform a Kegel without engaging or coordinating the rest of that system, you are strengthening one wall of a room while leaving the other three unaddressed. The room does not become stronger overall. One wall simply works harder to compensate.

Here is a concrete example. Imagine you are walking to the bathroom with urgency and you try to hold on by squeezing your pelvic floor muscles as hard as you can. For some women, that works. For others, the urgency gets worse, or the effort itself causes leakage. What is happening in the second case is that the pelvic floor is contracting under pressure from above, pressure that the diaphragm is creating with every breath and that the abdominals are not managing properly. The squeeze cannot override the pressure because the system sending the pressure downward is not being addressed.

There is also the matter of the tight floor, which was covered in Chapter 1. A pelvic floor that is already in a state of chronic contraction does not benefit from more contraction. Adding Kegels to an already overactive pelvic floor can increase tension, worsen urgency, and in some cases contribute to pelvic discomfort. The missing link for these women is not strength training. It is coordination and release. This chapter, and the exercises that follow in Chapters 5 through 8, address both patterns.

How Posture, Breathing, and Core Work Together

Think of a thermos. A well-made thermos maintains its internal environment because every part of its structure is doing its job: the walls, the lid, the base, all working together to keep pressure and temperature stable inside. Your core works on a similar principle. The diaphragm at the top, the pelvic floor at the base, the deep abdominal muscles at the front, and the lower back muscles at the rear form a sealed pressure system that manages the forces your body generates and absorbs every single day.

When you breathe in, your diaphragm drops downward into the abdominal cavity. That movement increases pressure inside the core canister. In a well-coordinated system, the pelvic floor responds by lengthening slightly to accommodate that pressure, and the abdominals and lower back muscles maintain the integrity of the walls so the load is distributed evenly. When you breathe out, the diaphragm rises, pressure decreases, and the pelvic floor gently recoils upward to its resting position. This exchange happens thousands of times a day without conscious effort.

What disrupts it is when one part of the system stops contributing. If your posture has shifted over the years into a forward-rounded position, the diaphragm cannot drop fully, breathing becomes shallow and chest-driven, and the pelvic floor receives inconsistent pressure signals. If your deep abdominal muscles are underactive, the front wall of the canister is soft and the pressure generated by breathing and movement leaks forward instead of being managed evenly. The pelvic floor then absorbs disproportionate downward load because the system above it is not holding its share.

Posture plays a more direct role than most people realize. A pelvis that tilts forward, a very common pattern in women who have spent years sitting at a desk or driving, places the pelvic floor muscles in a lengthened and weakened position. A pelvis that tucks under, equally common, compresses the floor and limits its range of motion. Neither position is neutral, and neither allows the pelvic floor to work the way it is designed to. The seated and standing posture checks in Chapter 3 address this directly.

Breath-holding during exertion is another common pattern that disrupts the system. Many women hold their breath when lifting, reaching, getting up from a chair, or doing any effortful movement. That held breath spikes the internal pressure suddenly and delivers it straight to the pelvic floor without preparation. Over years, this pattern contributes to the kind of stress leakage that seems to happen on impact: picking up a heavy bag, getting up quickly, or being caught off guard by a sneeze. Learning to exhale on the effort, which Chapter 3 covers in detail, is one of the most immediate and practical changes you can make.

The Muscle Groups You Must Train Together

You do not need to memorize anatomy to use this book effectively. But you do need to understand three things, because the entire program is built around training them as a unit.

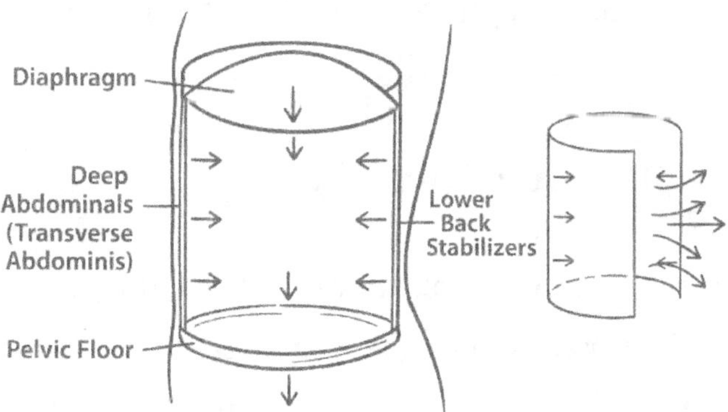

The breathing muscle. This is your diaphragm, and it is the engine of the whole system. How you breathe determines the pressure your pelvic floor has to manage on every repetition of every exercise. Getting your breathing pattern right first is not optional preparation. It is the foundation that makes everything else work. Chapter 3 teaches you how to do this before you attempt a single exercise.

The deep belly muscle. This is your transverse abdominis, a deep horizontal muscle that wraps around your midsection like a wide internal belt. In a healthy, well-coordinated core, this muscle activates automatically a fraction of a second before any movement you make. It braces the front wall of the canister so that pressure is distributed safely rather than dumped on the pelvic floor. After 60, and particularly for women who have had children, this muscle tends to become underactive. It stops firing first and lets the more superficial muscles take over. The foundation and strengthening exercises in Chapters 5 and 6 specifically retrain this coordination pattern.

The pelvic floor itself. Not just the squeeze, but the release. A pelvic floor that contracts well but cannot let go fully is not a healthy pelvic floor. It is a tense one. Training the pelvic floor means training both the lift and the release, the contraction and the relaxation, with equal attention given to each direction. The Reverse Kegel in Chapter 5 exists for exactly this reason, and it is the exercise that most books either skip entirely or mention briefly without teaching properly.

When these three groups are trained together with consistent breath coordination, the results accumulate differently than they do with isolated Kegel practice. The whole system becomes more responsive, more efficient, and more capable of handling the kinds of real-life pressure events that cause leakage and urgency. That is the difference this program is designed to deliver.

When to Check In with Your Doctor

Before starting this or any exercise program, there are specific situations where a brief conversation with your doctor or healthcare provider is the right first step. This is not a reason to delay indefinitely. It is a responsible starting point that protects your progress.

Check with your doctor before beginning if any of the following applies to you: you have been diagnosed with pelvic organ prolapse and have not yet discussed exercise with a specialist; you have had pelvic, abdominal, or spinal surgery within the past twelve weeks; you are currently experiencing significant pelvic pain or pressure at rest; you have an active urinary tract infection; you have unexplained bleeding; or you have been advised by a healthcare provider to restrict physical activity for any reason. In most cases, a brief consultation results in clearance to begin, sometimes with minor modifications. Knowing your starting point with that context makes the program more targeted and more effective.

If You Are Already Working with a Specialist

If you have previously seen or are currently seeing a pelvic floor physical therapist, everything in this program is compatible with that work. In fact, many of the exercises here align closely with standard clinical recommendations. If your therapist has given you specific guidelines, follow them. Use this program as a complement to that guidance, not a replacement for it.

The exercise chapters that follow are built on the principles this chapter has introduced. They train the breathing muscle, the deep belly muscle, and the pelvic floor together, in a sequence designed to build coordination before strength, and strength before endurance. That is the approach that produces results which hold beyond the four weeks of the program. Chapter 3 is where the practical work begins.

Part II: Build Your Foundation

Chapter 3

Breath and Body Awareness

Strength built on poor awareness is strength that misfires. Before you do a single Kegel, before you attempt a bridge or a pelvic tilt, you need to know how to breathe correctly and how to find the muscles you are about to train. These are not warm-up tasks. They are the actual foundation, and every exercise in this book becomes more effective the moment you have them in place.

How to Breathe Correctly During Exercise

Most adults breathe from their chest. You can verify this for yourself right now. Sit upright, place one hand on your chest and one hand on your belly, and take a normal breath. If the hand on your chest rises first and your belly stays relatively still, you are a chest breather. This is extremely common and, for general daily life, not a problem. For pelvic floor exercise, it is a significant limitation.

Diaphragmatic breathing, also called belly breathing, works differently. When you breathe in this way, the diaphragm drops downward into the abdominal cavity rather than the chest expanding outward and upward. The belly rises gently on the inhale as the organs below the diaphragm make room for it, and the belly falls on the exhale as the diaphragm returns to its resting dome shape. This breathing pattern creates the natural pressure rhythm that your pelvic floor is designed to work with.

Here is a simple test you can do right now, sitting in your chair. Sit tall with both feet flat on the floor. Place one hand lightly on your lower belly, just below your navel. Take a slow, easy breath in through your nose and direct that breath downward into your belly rather than upward into your chest. You should feel your hand rise gently. Hold for a moment, then breathe out slowly through your mouth and feel your hand lower. If your belly does not move at first, try placing both hands on your lower ribcage and breathing into your hands. The ribs should expand sideways on the inhale. With a little practice, this pattern becomes automatic during exercise.

Why does this matter specifically for pelvic floor work? Because the pelvic floor is meant to lengthen gently on the inhale and recoil on the exhale. When you breathe from your chest, the diaphragm does not drop, and the pelvic floor receives no rhythmic pressure signal. Worse, many chest breathers unconsciously hold their breath during effort, which creates sudden internal pressure spikes that the pelvic floor absorbs without warning. Learning to exhale during the effort part of any exercise, the lift, the squeeze, the push, is one of the most practical changes you can make, and it produces noticeable results quickly.

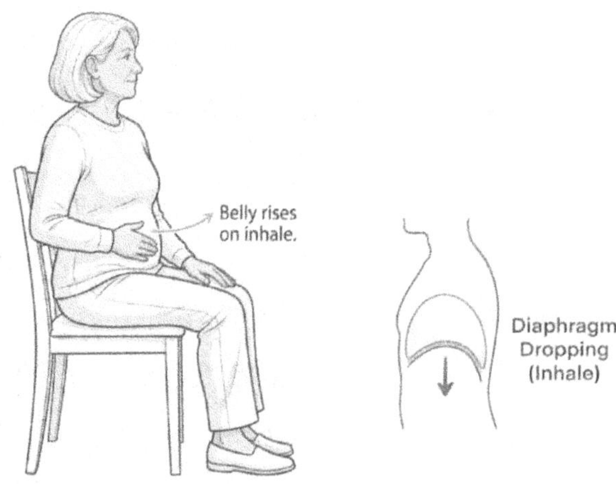

Finding and Feeling Your Pelvic Floor Muscles

This is the part of the chapter that makes some women feel slightly self-conscious, and that is completely understandable. Most of us have spent decades not thinking about these muscles deliberately. Being asked to locate them and engage them voluntarily can feel strange at first, particularly because there is no visible movement to confirm you are doing it correctly. That is normal. It takes a little practice, and the awkwardness passes quickly.

The first method for locating these muscles is the stop-flow method. The next time you visit the bathroom, briefly try to slow or stop the flow of urine midstream. The muscles you use to do that are part of your pelvic floor. Do not make this a regular habit or a form of exercise, as repeatedly stopping flow can interfere with bladder training. Use it once or twice simply to identify the sensation of the muscle engaging, then take that sensation with you to your chair for your actual practice.

The second method works seated. Sit upright on a firm chair with your feet flat on the floor and your weight evenly distributed across both sitting bones. Relax your thighs, your buttocks, and your abdomen completely. Now imagine you are trying to stop yourself from passing gas. The muscles you tighten to do that, drawing slightly inward and upward, are your pelvic floor. Hold gently for two seconds and then let go completely. The release is as important as the contraction. You should feel a clear difference between the two.

The most common mistake is recruiting the wrong muscles. Many women tighten their buttocks, squeeze their thighs together, or hold their breath during what they believe is a Kegel. None of those are pelvic floor contractions. The movement is internal and subtle. There should be no visible change in your posture, your leg position, or your breathing when you engage correctly. If you are unsure, pressing your fingers gently against your inner thighs will help you notice if you are inadvertently gripping there. A correctly performed contraction involves no thigh tension at all. The sensation is a gentle internal lift, as though the base of your pelvis is drawing upward and inward.

Seated Posture Check

Before any exercise session, taking thirty seconds to set up your seated posture pays dividends across every repetition that follows. Posture affects how pressure moves through your core, and a poorly aligned seated position puts the pelvic floor at a mechanical disadvantage before you even begin.

Start from the ground up. Place both feet flat on the floor, hip-width apart, with your weight distributed evenly across the full surface of each foot. Your knees should sit at approximately a 90-degree angle. If the chair is too high and your feet do not reach the floor easily, place a folded blanket or a firm cushion under them. Sit toward the front half of the chair rather than leaning back against the backrest. You want to feel your weight on your sitting bones, the two bony points at the base of your pelvis, rather than sinking into your tailbone.

From there, lengthen your spine upward without forcing it rigid. Think of stacking your vertebrae gently one on top of the other rather than pulling your shoulders back militarily.

Let your shoulders drop naturally away from your ears. Your chin should be level with the floor, not pushed forward or tucked tightly back. Your lower back should have a gentle natural curve, not a pronounced arch and not flattened entirely. From this position, take a slow breath in through your nose and feel your belly expand. This is the foundation position for every seated exercise in this book.

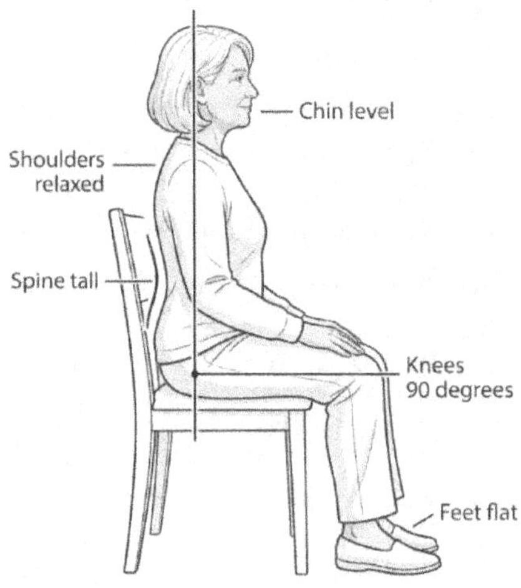

Standing Posture Check

Correct standing posture matters for the same reason correct seated posture does: it places your pelvic floor in a neutral, functional position where it can respond to load efficiently. Many women develop a standing posture over the years that tilts the pelvis forward, which lengthens and weakens the pelvic floor muscles, or backward, which compresses them and limits their range. Neither position is where you want to begin an exercise.

Stand with your feet hip-width apart and your weight distributed evenly across both feet, from heel to toe on each side. Soften your knees very slightly, enough to unlock them without bending them noticeably. Gently draw your lower belly inward and upward, a light engagement of the deep abdominal muscles without gripping or sucking in aggressively. Let your pelvis find its neutral position: not tilted forward into an exaggerated lower back arch, and not tucked under. Your tailbone should point toward the floor. Your spine should feel long, your shoulders relaxed and wide, your head balanced easily on top of your neck without pushing forward.

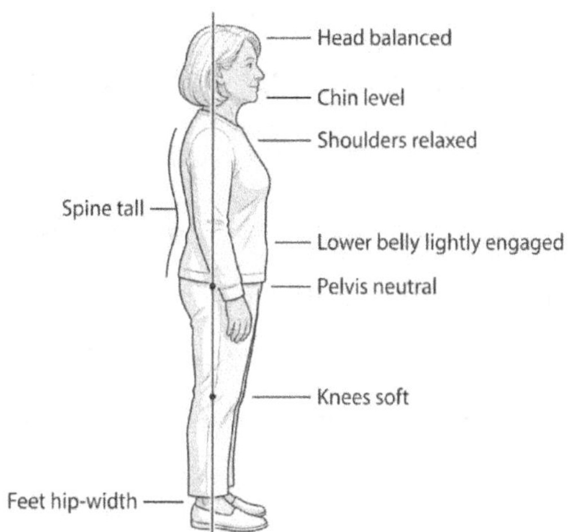

These four skills, diaphragmatic breathing, pelvic floor awareness, correct seated alignment, and correct standing alignment, are the foundation beneath every exercise that follows. You do not need to master them perfectly before you begin the program. You simply need to bring your attention to them at the start of each session. Within a week, they will begin to feel habitual. Within two weeks, you will notice yourself applying them without thinking about it during your daily routine. That automatic awareness is exactly where you want to be when you get to the strengthening and bladder control work in Chapters 5 through 8.

Chapter 4

Warm-Up and Cool-Down Routines

Cold muscles and stiff joints do not respond well to exercise, and after 60, the warm-up is not optional prep work. It is the difference between a session that builds something and one that sets something back. The nine movements in this chapter take about ten minutes total and they are the starting point for every workout session in this book.

Why Warm-Ups Matter More After 60

Joint fluid, the synovial fluid that cushions your knees, hips, and ankles, does not circulate well when you are sitting still. It thickens slightly at rest and takes several minutes of gentle movement to thin out and spread evenly across the joint surfaces. Moving into any strengthening exercise without first warming those joints up is like trying to open a stiff hinge without oiling it. The resistance is unnecessary and the risk of irritation is real.

Muscle tissue also changes with age. Younger muscle fibers have more elasticity and recover quickly from the initial demand of exercise. Older muscle needs more time to increase blood flow and reach the temperature at which it contracts and releases most efficiently. A five- to ten-minute warm-up raises your core muscle temperature by one to two degrees, and that change alone improves both strength output and coordination during the workout that follows.

Circulation is the third reason this matters. During rest, blood pools toward the core and the major organs. Gentle rhythmic movement redirects blood flow toward the working muscles, bringing oxygen and clearing the byproducts of metabolism. For women managing blood pressure changes or circulation issues that often come with age, this gradual increase is also safer than a cold start into any demanding movement.

Warm-Up Exercises

1. Seated Ankle Circles

This gentle movement wakes up the ankle joints and begins the circulation process in your lower legs before you place any weight-bearing demand on your feet.

Starting Position:

Sit upright on a firm chair with both feet flat on the floor, hip-width apart.

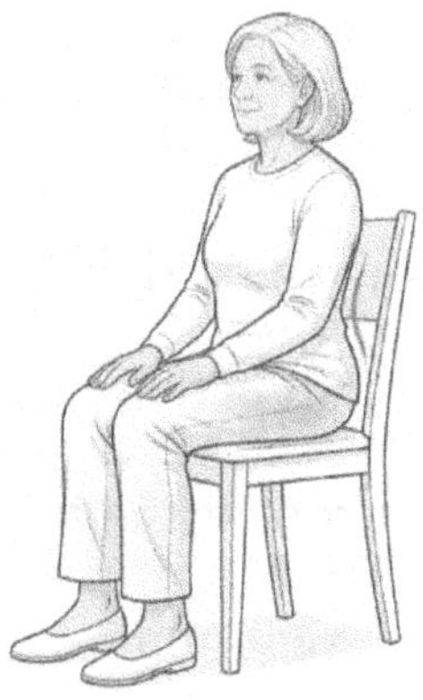

Steps:
1. Shift your weight slightly to your left sitting bone then lift your right foot one inch off the floor.

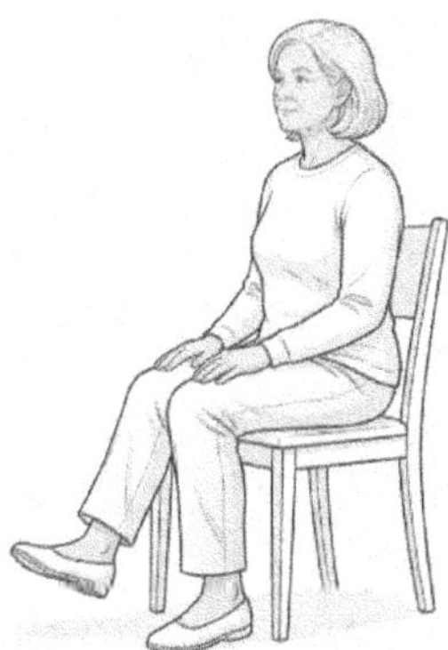

2. Slowly rotate your foot in a full circle to the right, tracing the largest circle you can.

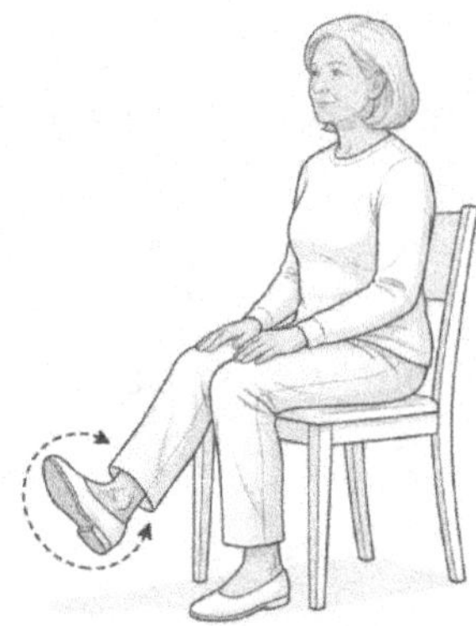

3. Complete five full circles, moving slowly and deliberately.

4. Pause, then reverse the direction and circle five times to the left.

5. Lower your right foot to the floor and repeat the full sequence on your left foot.

Reps / Hold: 5 circles in each direction per ankle
Sets: 2 sets per ankle

If this feels difficult: If lifting your foot causes hip discomfort, keep your heel on the floor and draw the circles with just your toes, lifting only the forefoot.

Why this works: Ankle circulation feeds directly into pelvic floor health because poor lower-leg blood flow adds to the pelvic congestion that worsens heaviness and pressure symptoms. Starting here creates a gentle bottom-up blood flow before any core work begins.

2. Seated Knee Lifts

Seated knee lifts activate the hip flexors and wake up the deep abdominals that connect to the pelvic floor, giving your core system a low-demand first signal before the exercises that follow.

Starting Position:

Sit upright toward the front half of your chair with both feet flat on the floor, hip-width apart. Rest your hands lightly on your thighs. Lengthen your spine without forcing your lower back into a rigid arch.

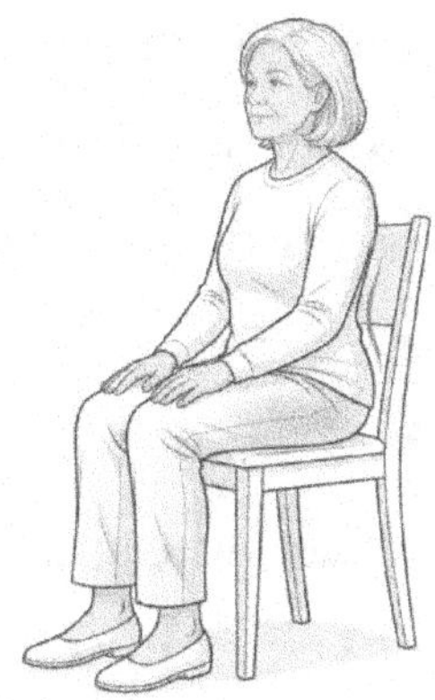

Steps:

1. Breathe in slowly and let your belly relax.

2. As you breathe out, gently draw your lower belly inward and lift your right knee toward the ceiling.

3. Lift until your thigh is parallel to the floor or as high as is comfortable without leaning back.

4. Hold the lifted position for two seconds, keeping your breathing steady.

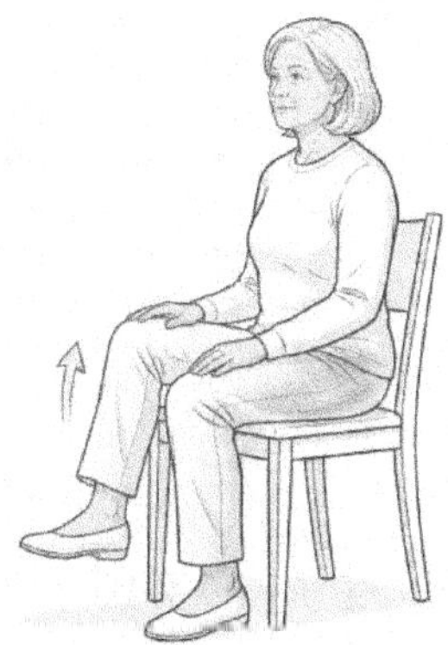

5. Lower your right foot slowly back to the floor as you breathe in.

6. Repeat the lift on your left side. That is one full repetition.

Reps / Hold: 10 repetitions alternating sides
Sets: 2 sets

If this feels difficult: If lifting the full thigh is uncomfortable, begin by simply sliding one heel backward under the chair and lifting only the heel off the floor while keeping the toe down. This activates the same hip flexor muscles with far less range of motion.

Why this works: The hip flexors and the pelvic floor share connective tissue pathways. When the hip flexors are underactive, the pelvic floor compensates for instability. This exercise wakes up that connection before any direct pelvic floor work begins.

3. Seated Torso Rotation

Gentle rotation through the mid-back releases the spinal stiffness that accumulates from prolonged sitting and prepares the lower back and core to work through their full range during the exercises ahead.

Starting Position:

Sit upright on a firm chair with both feet flat on the floor, hip-width apart. Cross your arms loosely over your chest or rest your hands on your shoulders. Sit tall and let your lower back find its natural gentle curve.

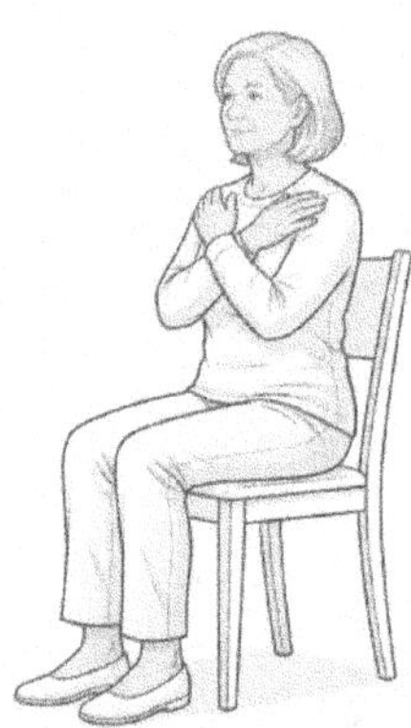

Steps:
1. Breathe in to prepare, sitting as tall as you can without straining.

2. As you breathe out, slowly rotate your upper body to the right, leading with your right shoulder.

3. Rotate only as far as feels comfortable, keeping your hips and knees facing forward throughout.

4. Hold the rotated position for two seconds and breathe in.

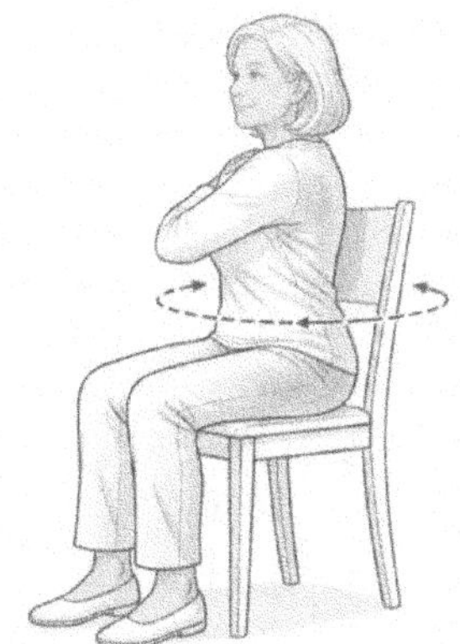

5. As you breathe out, slowly rotate back through center and continue to the left side.

6. Hold the left rotation for two seconds, then return to center. That is one full repetition.

Reps / Hold: 8 full rotations, alternating right and left
Sets: 2 sets

If this feels difficult: If your range of motion is limited, reduce the rotation to whatever is comfortable and focus on the feeling of length through the spine rather than the degree of the turn. The movement does not need to be large to be effective.

Why this works: The thoracic spine and lower back share load management with the pelvic floor. When the mid-back is stiff, the lumbar spine and pelvis compensate, placing extra demand on the pelvic floor muscles. This rotation helps free that connection before any direct core work.

4. Seated Hip Circles

Hip circles warm up the hip joint capsule and the muscles that wrap around it, including the deep hip rotators that sit adjacent to the pelvic floor and directly influence how well it functions.

Starting Position:

Sit upright near the front edge of your chair with both feet flat on the floor, hip-width apart. Rest your hands on your thighs for light support. Your spine is tall and your weight is on both sitting bones equally.

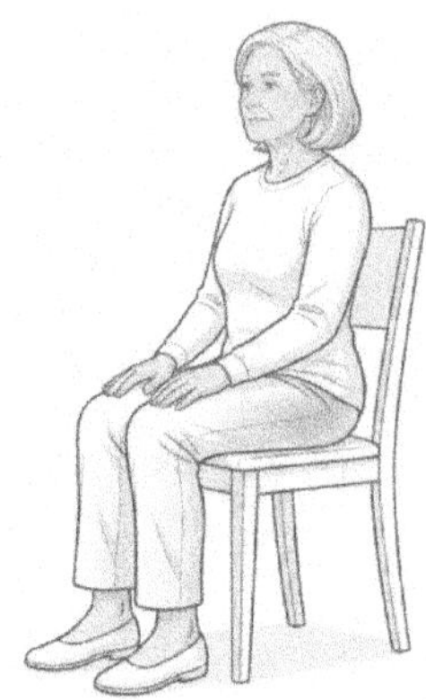

Steps:

1. Breathe in and sit as tall as possible, lengthening your spine upward.

2. Begin to tilt your pelvis slightly forward, letting your lower back gently arch.

3. Continue circling to the right, shifting your weight toward your right sitting bone.

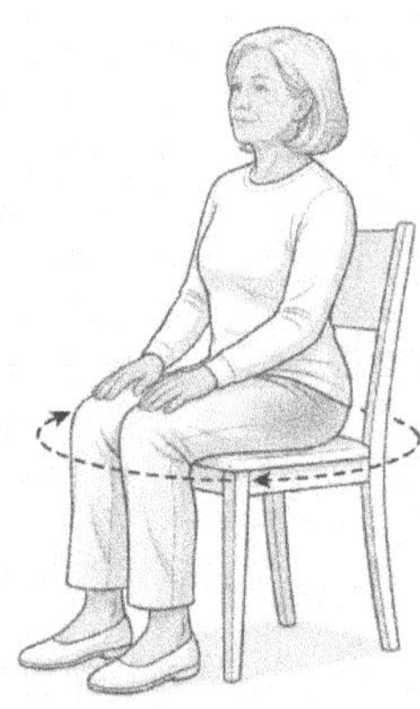

4. Roll through the back of your pelvis, tucking your tailbone slightly under, then shift to the left sitting bone.

5. Complete the circle by returning to the forward tilt and back to center.

6. Complete 5 full clockwise circles, then reverse and complete 5 counter-clockwise.

Reps / Hold: 5 circles in each direction
Sets: 2 sets

If this feels difficult: If the full circular motion causes discomfort, simplify it to a forward-and-back pelvic rock only. Rock your pelvis forward into a gentle arch, then back into a gentle tuck, ten times. This delivers the same joint lubrication benefit with a smaller range of motion.

Why this works: The deep hip rotators and the pelvic floor are anatomical neighbors. Stiffness in one creates compensation in the other. Warming the hip joint through its full range before exercise reduces the demand placed on the pelvic floor muscles to stabilize around a restricted joint.

5. Shoulder Rolls and Neck Release

Upper body tension travels downward through the spine into the lower back and pelvis. Releasing the shoulders and neck before pelvic floor work ensures you are not carrying unnecessary tension into exercises that require your whole body to be as relaxed as possible.

Starting Position:

Sit upright on your chair with both feet flat on the floor. Let your arms rest loosely at your sides or in your lap. Lengthen your spine and let your chin drop very slightly so the back of your neck feels long.

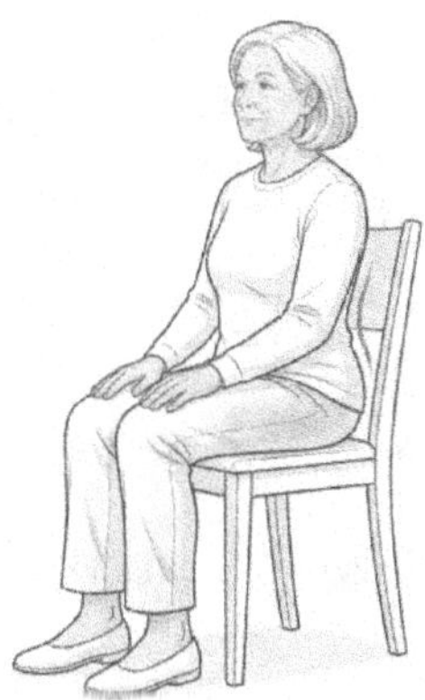

Steps:
1. Breathe in and draw both shoulders upward toward your ears.

2. Roll both shoulders backward in a large slow circle, squeezing the shoulder blades together at the back.

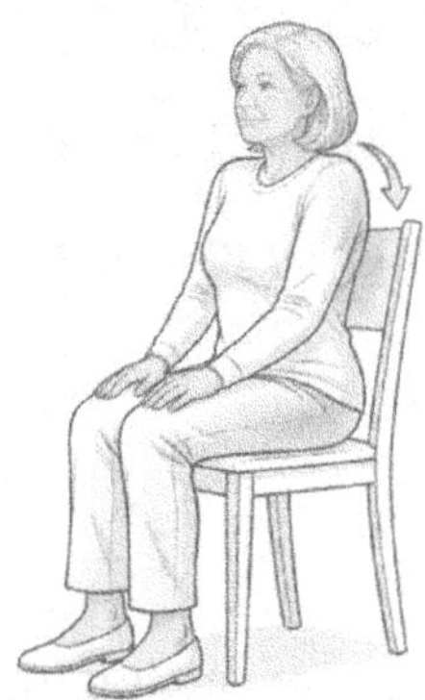

3. Continue the circle, dropping the shoulders down and forward, then returning to the starting position.

4. Complete 5 full backward circles, then reverse and complete 5 forward circles.

5. After the shoulder circles, return to sitting tall and gently tilt your head to the right, ear toward shoulder.

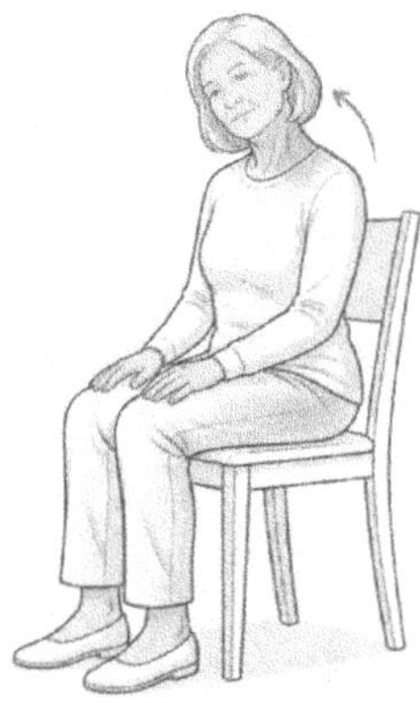

6. Hold for five slow breaths, then lift your head back to center and repeat on the left side.

Reps / Hold: 5 shoulder circles each direction, then 5-breath hold each side for neck
Sets: 1 set

If this feels difficult: If rolling the shoulders causes any clicking or discomfort in the shoulder joint, reduce the circle to a simple shrug up and release down, repeated ten times. For the neck, reduce the tilt to a very small movement and focus on breathing into the stretch rather than increasing the range.

Why this works: Chronic tension held in the shoulders and upper neck braces the entire spine, including the lower back and pelvic region. Releasing this tension before pelvic floor work allows the diaphragm to drop freely on each inhale, which directly supports the pelvic floor coordination you are about to train.

The five warm-up movements above should take between eight and twelve minutes at a comfortable pace. Do not rush through them. By the time you complete the shoulder and neck release, your joints are lubricated, your circulation has increased, your core temperature has risen slightly, and your body is ready to work. The cool-down sequences below serve the opposite function. They bring your system back down gently after exercise and, importantly, they include the one step that most pelvic floor books skip entirely.

Cool-Down and Release Stretches

6. Seated Forward Fold

The seated forward fold gently decompresses the lower spine and begins to release the tension that builds in the hamstrings and lower back during any exercise session. It is also a natural cue to the nervous system that the demanding work is done.

Starting Position:

Sit upright near the front edge of your chair with both feet flat on the floor, slightly wider than hip-width apart and parallel to each other. Rest your hands on your thighs.

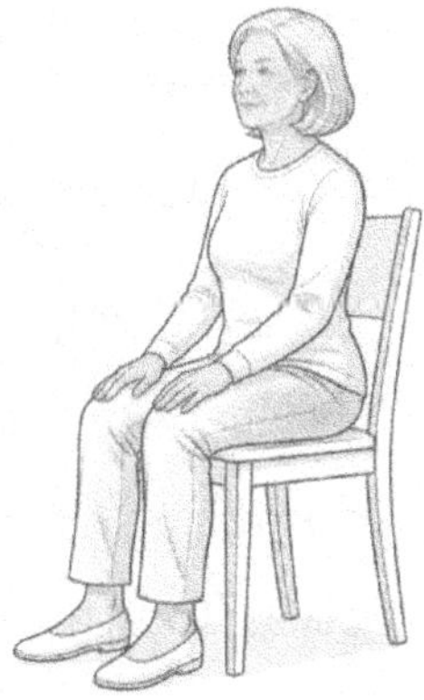

Steps:

1. Breathe in and sit as tall as you can, lengthening through the crown of your head.

2. As you breathe out, hinge forward from your hips, not from your waist, letting your chest move toward your thighs.

3. Allow your hands to slide down your shins (the front of your legs below the knee) or toward the floor, resting wherever they reach comfortably.

4. Let your head hang gently and release any tension in your neck and shoulders.

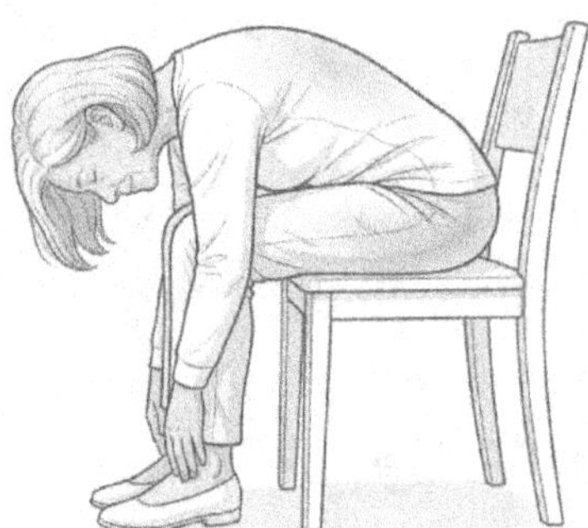

5. Hold this position and breathe slowly, allowing the fold to deepen slightly with each exhale.

6. To come up, breathe in and slowly roll back to seated, stacking the spine one vertebra at a time.

Reps / Hold: Hold for 5 to 8 slow breaths
Sets: 2 sets

If this feels difficult: If hinging forward causes lower back discomfort, place a folded blanket under your sitting bones to tilt the pelvis forward slightly before you fold. If reaching toward your shins is uncomfortable, rest your forearms on your thighs instead and simply allow your chest to lower toward your legs without reaching.

Why this works: Forward folding after exercise helps the erector spinae muscles of the lower back, which work alongside the pelvic floor during every standing and seated exercise, to lengthen and release. This decompression reduces the residual tension that, if left unchecked, gradually tightens the pelvic floor muscles between sessions.

7. Supine Knees to Chest

This floor-based stretch gently decompresses the sacrum and lower lumbar spine, releasing the deep postural muscles that hold tension throughout the day and directly influence pelvic floor position.

Starting Position:

Lie on your back on a firm, comfortable surface such as a yoga mat or carpeted floor. Extend both legs out straight with your arms resting at your sides, palms facing downward. Take two slow breaths before beginning.

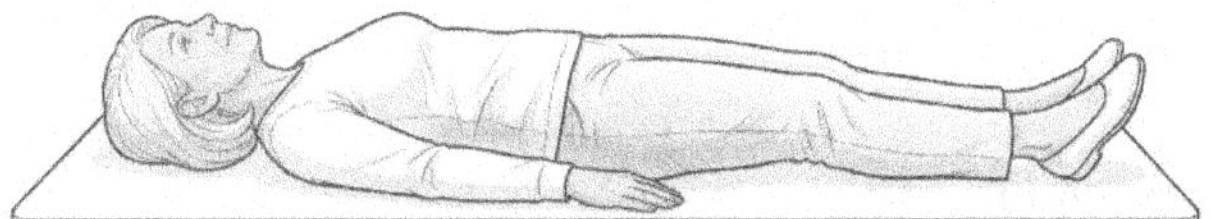

Steps:

1. Breathe in, and as you breathe out, draw both knees slowly toward your chest.

2. Wrap your hands around your shins just below your knees, one hand on each shin.

3. Gently draw your knees closer to your chest until you feel a comfortable stretch across your lower back and sacrum.

4. Hold the position and breathe slowly and fully, letting your lower back soften into the mat on each exhale.

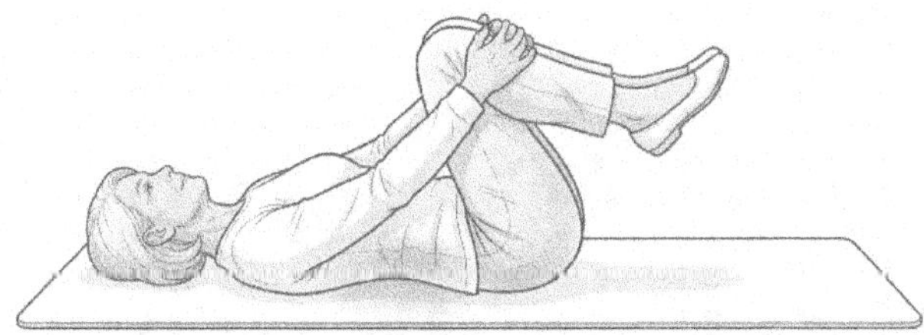

5. After holding, gently rock from side to side, just an inch or two each way, to massage the sacrum.

6. Release by slowly lowering both feet back to the floor, one at a time.

Reps / Hold: Hold for 20 to 30 seconds, then rock gently for 10 seconds
Sets: 2 sets

If this feels difficult: If getting down to the floor is difficult or uncomfortable, this stretch can be adapted in the chair. Sit toward the front edge of your chair, then slowly draw one knee up toward your chest with both hands and hold for 20 seconds before switching sides. This delivers a similar sacral release effect without requiring floor work.

Why this works: The sacrum is the attachment point for several of the pelvic floor muscles. When the sacrum is compressed and the surrounding muscles are tight from prolonged sitting or exercise, the pelvic floor has less room to move through its full range. This stretch creates space and helps the pelvic floor muscles return to their resting length after a workout.

8. Pelvic Floor Release Stretch

This is the exercise that most pelvic floor books skip, and it may be the most important cool-down movement in this entire chapter. Strengthening work contracts the pelvic floor muscles repeatedly. Without a deliberate release at the end of every session, those muscles gradually accumulate tension that compounds over days and weeks. Learning to fully relax the pelvic floor after exercise is as important as the exercise itself.

Starting Position:

Lie on your back on a firm mat with your knees bent and your feet flat on the floor, hip-width apart. Place one hand lightly on your lower belly and let the other rest at your side. Take three slow, full diaphragmatic breaths before beginning.

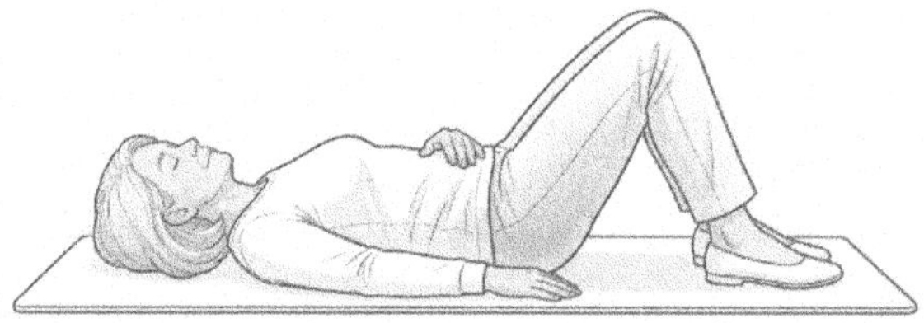

Steps:
1. Close your eyes and bring your attention to the area between your sitting bones.

2. Breathe in slowly through your nose, directing the breath downward into your belly. Feel your hand rise.

3. As you breathe in, consciously let your pelvic floor muscles go. Imagine them softening and widening, like a fist very slowly opening.

4. Do not push down. The release is a letting go, not an effort. Simply allow the muscles to stop holding.

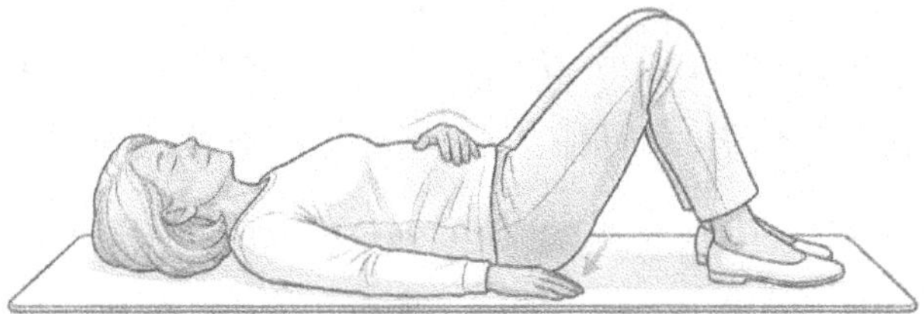

5. Hold the released, open state for a full five-second breath, then gently breathe out and allow the pelvic floor to naturally return to its resting tone.

6. Repeat the cycle: breathe in and release fully, hold for five seconds, breathe out and return to resting tone.

Reps / Hold: 6 to 8 full breath cycles of conscious release
Sets: 1 set, performed slowly and without rushing

If this feels difficult: If you find it difficult to feel the release, try the following: during your inhale, gently part your knees slightly wider, allowing gravity to help open the inner thighs and create more space at the base of the pelvis. Some women find this positional cue makes the release sensation much easier to access initially.

Why this works: A pelvic floor that cannot release fully is a pelvic floor that is always bracing. Chronic bracing leads to tightness, urgency, incomplete emptying, and discomfort. The purpose of this exercise is not stretching in the traditional sense. It is neuromuscular training for the release direction, teaching the pelvic floor muscles the same deliberate control in the letting-go phase that the Kegel exercises train in the contraction phase. Both directions of control matter equally.

Why the Release Matters as Much as the Strengthening

Most pelvic floor programs focus entirely on contraction. The assumption is that a stronger pelvic floor is always better. That is only half true. A healthy pelvic floor needs to be able to contract firmly when you need it to and release completely when it does not need to be working. When the release is missing from a program, the muscles get stronger but also tighter. For women with an already overactive pelvic floor, this worsens symptoms rather than improving them. This is why the Pelvic Floor Release Stretch closes every session in this program, not because it is a nice-to-do but because it is the completion of the work you have done.

Take your time here. This is the one movement in the program where slower is always better.

Part III: The Illustrated Workout Library

A Quick Favor – Before the Workout Library

You are halfway through.

The foundation is built. You understand your body better than you did when you opened this book. You have found the muscles, learned the breathing, and started the work.

If what you have read so far has been useful, there is one small thing that would mean a great deal.

Leave a review on Amazon.

This book has no publishing house behind it, no marketing team, no advertising budget. What it has is readers like you, and your honest words carry more weight than any campaign ever could. A sentence or two is enough. It helps other women find guidance they have been quietly looking for. It helps daughters and caregivers find something genuinely useful for the women they love. It helps this book reach the hands it was made for.

Search the title on Amazon. It takes two minutes, and it matters more than you know.

Now, back to the work. Chapter 5 is where things start to come together.

Chapter 5

Foundation Exercises — Awareness and Control

Every exercise in the chapters ahead depends on the five movements in this chapter. Not because they are simple, though they are, but because they train the specific muscle coordination that makes the harder work effective. Do not skip this chapter, even if you have done Kegels before.

Chapter 2 introduced the whole-system approach: the diaphragm, the deep abdominals, the lower back, and the pelvic floor all working as one coordinated unit. These five exercises are where that coordination begins. Each one targets a specific part of the system. By the time you have worked through all five consistently in Week 1 of the program, your body will begin to connect these parts automatically, and you will feel that integration carrying over into the strengthening exercises in Chapter 6.

Foundation Exercises

1. Basic Kegel

This is the starting point for pelvic floor training, and it is also the exercise most women think they know how to do but often perform incorrectly. Getting the technique right here changes everything that follows.

Starting Position:

Sit upright on a firm chair with both feet flat on the floor, hip-width apart, and your hands resting lightly on your thighs. Your spine is tall, your shoulders are relaxed, and your jaw is unclenched.

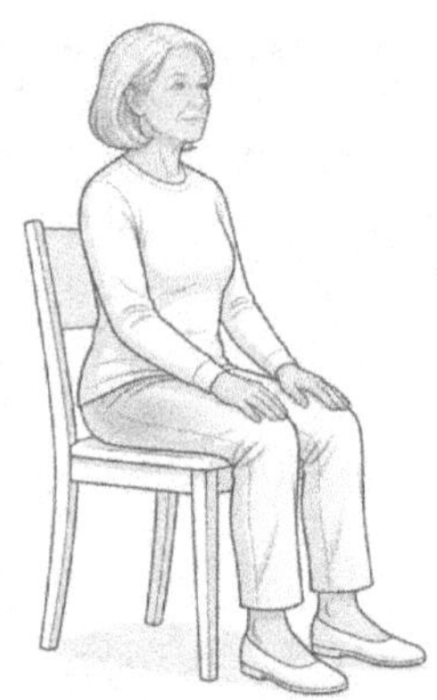

Steps:

1. Breathe in slowly through your nose and let your belly, thighs, and pelvic floor fully relax.

2. As you breathe out, gently lift and squeeze the muscles around your urethra and vagina, as though stopping the flow of urine.

3. Hold the lift for five seconds, breathing normally. Do not hold your breath.

4. Release slowly and completely over five seconds. The release is as deliberate as the contraction.

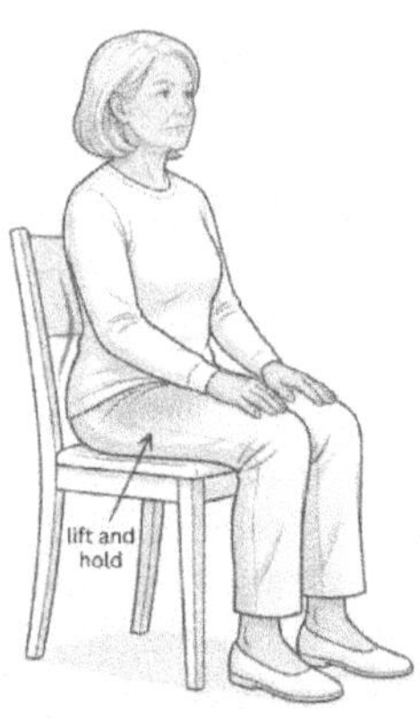

5. Rest for five seconds between each contraction. The rest is not optional.

6. Repeat the lift, hold, and release sequence ten times to complete one set.

Reps / Hold: 10 contractions, 5-second hold each
Sets: 3 sets, with a 60-second rest between sets

If this feels difficult: Begin with a 2-second hold and build toward 5 seconds over the first week. A shorter hold performed correctly is far more effective than a longer hold that recruits the wrong muscles.

Why this works: Each controlled contraction builds the endurance and fast-twitch response that prevents leakage during coughing, sneezing, and sudden movement. The relaxation phase prevents the chronic tension that worsens urgency over time.

Common Mistake: What Correct Feels Like

The most common Kegel error is tightening the buttocks, squeezing the thighs together, or bearing down instead of lifting up. If you notice any of those happening, stop, breathe, and start again. A correct Kegel involves only the internal muscles of the pelvic floor: a gentle lift upward and inward, with nothing changing visibly on the outside. Your breathing continues. Your face stays relaxed. Your thighs stay still. If you are unsure whether you are recruiting the right muscles, return to "Finding and Feeling Your Pelvic Floor Muscles" section in Chapter 3 before continuing.

2. Reverse Kegel

The Reverse Kegel is the deliberate, conscious release of the pelvic floor muscles. Most women have never been taught this movement, and most pelvic floor books do not include it. For women with a tight or overactive pelvic floor, it is more important than the Basic Kegel. For all women, it trains the release direction of pelvic floor control with the same intention that the contraction direction receives.

A pelvic floor that can only contract is like a hand that can only make a fist. Full function requires both directions. The Reverse Kegel teaches the muscles that it is safe to let go fully, which reduces chronic tension, may help with urgency, and is an essential preparation for the Diaphragmatic Breathing with Movement exercise that closes this chapter.

Starting Position:

Lie on your back on a firm mat with your knees bent and feet flat on the floor, hip-width apart. Place one hand on your lower belly. Let your entire body become heavy and still before you begin.

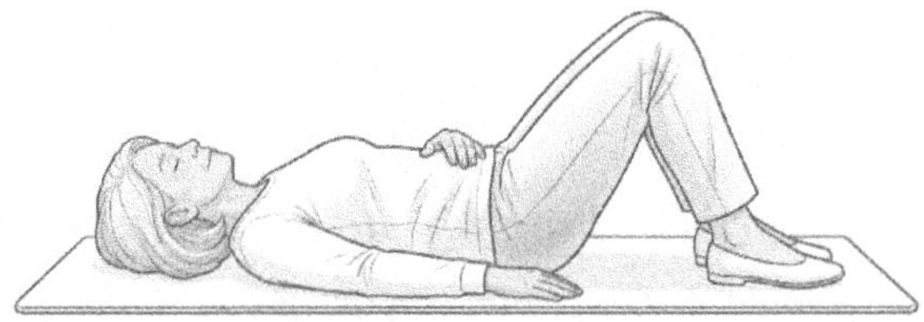

Steps:

1. Close your eyes and bring your attention to the base of your pelvis between your sitting bones.

2. Breathe in slowly through your nose, directing the breath downward into your belly. Feel your hand rise.

3. As you breathe in, consciously allow the pelvic floor to soften, widen, and drop. Imagine the muscles gently opening like a hand uncurling from a fist.

4. Hold this open, released state for a full three to five seconds while continuing to breathe slowly.

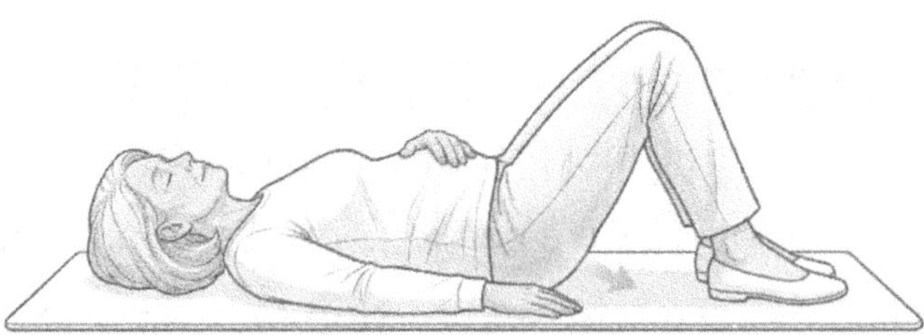

5. As you breathe out, allow the pelvic floor to naturally return to its resting tone without contracting it deliberately.

6. Pause for two seconds, then begin the next breath cycle and release. Repeat slowly and without rushing.

Reps / Hold: 6 to 8 slow breath cycles of conscious release
Sets: 2 sets

If this feels difficult: If you find it hard to locate the release sensation, try gently widening your knees two inches further apart during the inhale. The change in inner thigh position often makes the pelvic floor release easier to feel. Some women also find it helpful to first perform a brief Basic Kegel contraction and then deliberately let it go, using the contrast to identify both sensations clearly.

Why this works: For women with an overactive pelvic floor, this exercise directly addresses urgency, incomplete emptying, and pelvic discomfort by training the muscles to release tension rather than accumulate it. For all women, it completes the full range of pelvic floor control that the Basic Kegel alone cannot provide.

3. Pelvic Tilt

The Pelvic Tilt reactivates the deep abdominals and lower back stabilizers that work in coordination with the pelvic floor, restoring the neutral pelvis position that is the foundation for every load-bearing exercise in Chapter 6.

Starting Position:

Lie on your back on a firm mat with your knees bent and feet flat on the floor, hip-width apart. Rest both arms at your sides, palms facing down. Notice whether your lower back has a small natural arch off the mat, which is the neutral position you are working with.

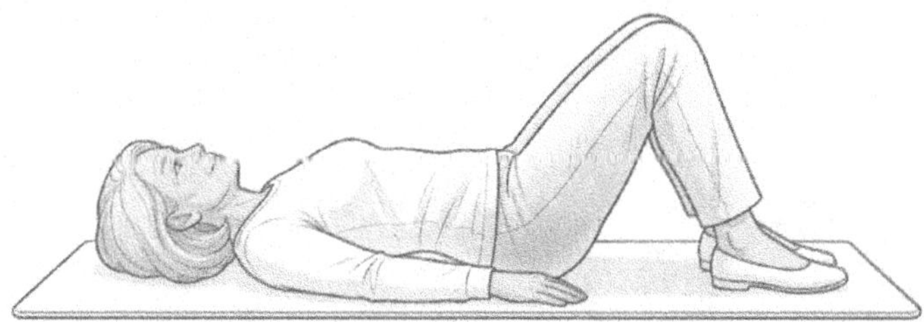

Steps:
1. Breathe in slowly and let your lower back and pelvis fully relax.
2. As you breathe out, gently draw your lower belly inward and tilt your pelvis so your lower back presses lightly toward the mat.

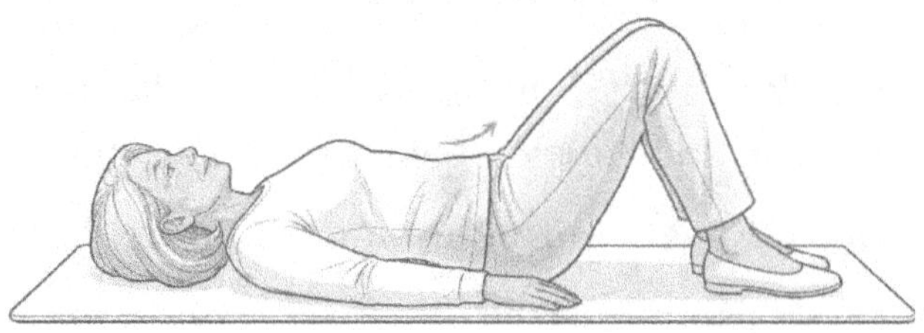

3. Hold the tilted position for three seconds. The movement is small. Your hips do not leave the mat.

4. Breathe in and slowly release, allowing the lower back to return to its natural arch.

5. Repeat the tilt and release in a slow, controlled rhythm.

6. Each tilt and release counts as one repetition.

Reps / Hold: 12 repetitions
Sets: 3 sets

If this feels difficult: If pressing your lower back to the mat causes discomfort, reduce the range to a very small movement, just enough to feel your lower abdominals engage lightly. The goal is muscle activation, not a specific amount of spinal movement.

Why this works: Neutral pelvis alignment is the position in which the pelvic floor muscles can generate their best force and coordination. When the pelvis habitually sits in a forward or backward tilt, the pelvic floor is mechanically disadvantaged before any exercise begins. This movement trains the awareness and muscle control needed to find and hold neutral.

4. Seated Core Engagement

This exercise trains the transverse abdominis, the deep belt-like abdominal muscle introduced in Chapter 2, to engage lightly and consistently before and during movement, which is exactly the role it plays in protecting the pelvic floor during daily activity.

Starting Position:

Sit upright on a firm chair with both feet flat on the floor, hip-width apart. Place one hand on your lower belly, just below your navel. Sit tall without rigidly holding your breath or gripping your abdominals.

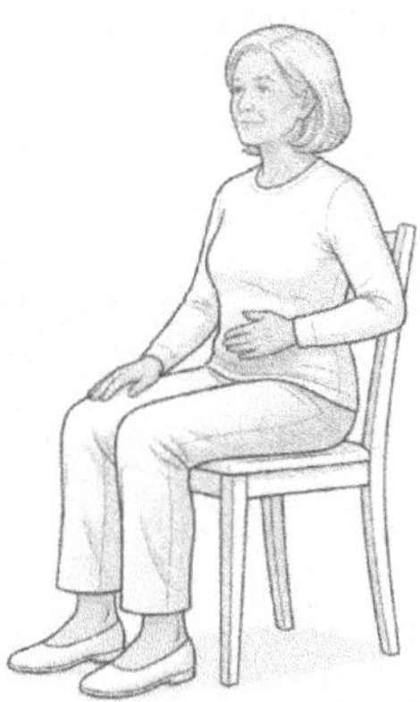

Steps:

1. Breathe in slowly and allow your belly to expand into your hand.

2. As you breathe out, draw your lower belly gently inward and upward, away from your waistband. Your hand should feel the belly pull lightly back.

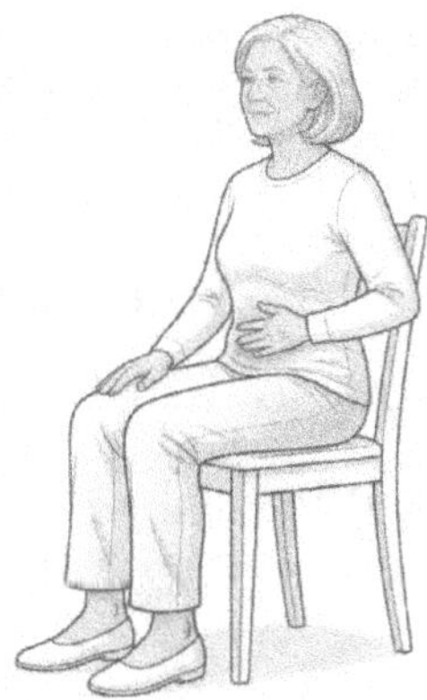

3. Hold this light engagement at about 30 percent of your maximum effort. This is not a full suck-in.

4. Continue breathing normally while maintaining the light engagement. Do not hold your breath.

5. Hold the light engagement for five seconds while taking two or three normal breaths.

6. Release fully and rest for five seconds before repeating.

Reps / Hold: 10 repetitions, 5-second hold each
Sets: 3 sets

If this feels difficult: If holding the engagement while breathing feels like too many things at once, start with just two breathing cycles per hold and build from there. The coordination of breathing and light abdominal engagement takes practice and does not need to arrive all at once.

Why this works: The transverse abdominis is designed to engage a fraction of a second before any movement your body makes. Training this anticipatory pattern seated makes it available during walking, lifting, and standing, reducing the unmanaged pressure load that reaches your pelvic floor throughout the day.

5. Diaphragmatic Breathing with Movement

This exercise brings together the breath, the pelvic floor, and the deep abdominals in a single coordinated movement. It is the clearest demonstration of the whole-system approach from Chapter 2 and the template for how breathing should work during every exercise in this program.

Starting Position:

Sit upright on a firm chair with both feet flat on the floor, hip-width apart. Place one hand on your lower belly and one hand on your lower ribcage at the side. Sit tall and breathe normally for several seconds before beginning.

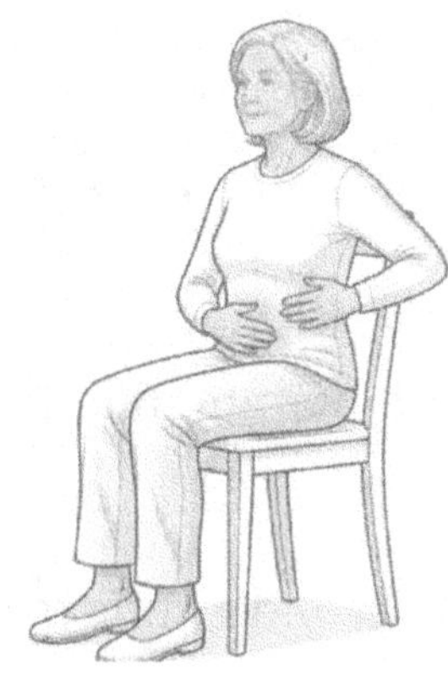

Steps:

1. Breathe in slowly through your nose, directing the breath into your belly and lower ribs. Both hands should rise and expand outward.

2. As you breathe in, consciously allow your pelvic floor to soften and gently drop. Do not force it down, simply permit the release.

3. Pause for one second at the top of the inhale.

4. As you breathe out through your mouth, gently draw your lower belly inward and allow the pelvic floor to lift naturally with the exhale.

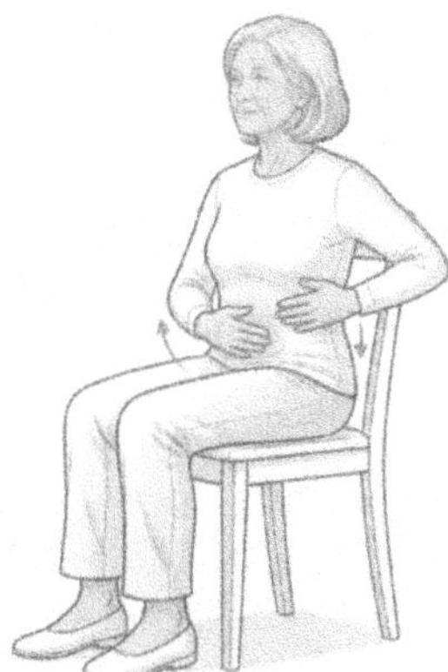

5. Complete the exhale fully, allowing the belly and pelvic floor to return without forcing either.

6. Pause for one second at the bottom of the exhale before beginning the next inhale. Repeat the full cycle.

Reps / Hold: 8 to 10 full breath cycles
Sets: 3 sets, with 30-second rest between sets

If this feels difficult: If coordinating the pelvic floor awareness with the breath feels too complex initially, separate the tasks. Spend the first week simply practicing the diaphragmatic breath until it feels natural. In the second week, add the pelvic floor awareness layer. Coordination between breath and pelvic floor emerges with repetition and does not need to be forced.

Why this works: This is the foundational breathing pattern used in every strengthening and bladder control exercise in this program. Training it in isolation now means you will not be thinking about your breath during the more demanding movements ahead. The coordination becomes automatic, and the results of every other exercise improve as a result.

Chapter 6

Strengthening Exercises — Building Core Strength

Standing up from a low chair. Carrying groceries from the car to the kitchen. Walking across a parking lot without bracing. These are the movements that tell you whether your core is doing its job, and they are exactly what the six exercises in this chapter are designed to support.

Core strength and pelvic floor health are not separate goals. The deep abdominals, the glutes, the hip stabilizers, and the pelvic floor all share load during every weight-bearing movement you make. When the core muscles surrounding the pelvic floor are strong and well-coordinated, the pelvic floor does not have to compensate for instability. It can do its own job, which is pressure management and continence, rather than spending its capacity propping up a weak surrounding system. The exercises here build that surrounding strength progressively, starting from the floor and working to standing.

Core Strength Exercises

1. Bridge

The bridge is the most direct floor-based exercise for building glute and hamstring strength while simultaneously training the pelvic floor to engage under load. It is the cornerstone of the strength section in this program.

Starting Position:

Lie on your back on a firm mat with your knees bent at approximately 90 degrees and your feet flat on the floor, hip-width apart. Rest your arms at your sides, palms facing down. Find your neutral lower back position before beginning.

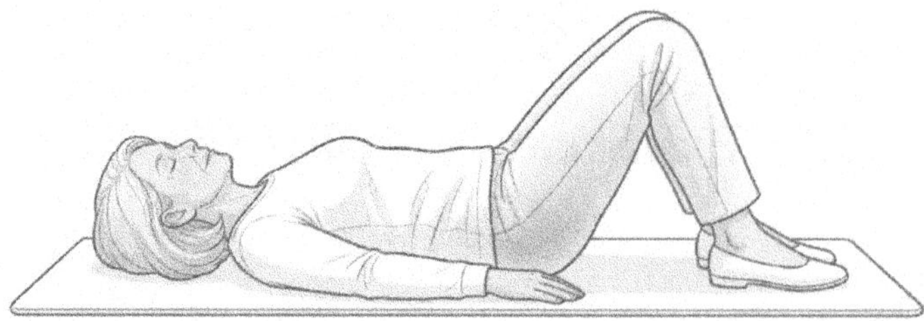

Steps:

1. Breathe in slowly and let your body settle into the mat.

2. As you breathe out, gently engage your lower belly, then press through both feet and lift your hips off the mat.

3. Lift until your body forms a straight diagonal line from your knees to your shoulders. Do not arch your lower back beyond this line.

4. Squeeze your glutes gently at the top and hold for three seconds, continuing to breathe.

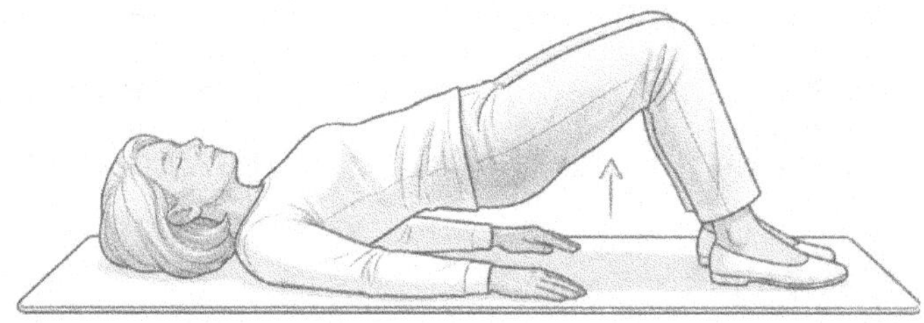

5. As you breathe in, slowly lower your hips back to the mat in a controlled movement. Do not drop.

6. Allow your lower back to return to neutral before beginning the next repetition.

Reps / Hold: 10 repetitions
Sets: 3 sets

If this feels difficult: If lifting the full hips is uncomfortable, begin with a smaller range of movement. Lift only enough to feel the glutes engage, even if the hips come only two or three inches off the mat. Build range gradually over the first week rather than forcing the full position immediately.

Why this works: The glutes and hamstrings act as the primary load carriers during standing and walking. When they are strong, the pelvic floor receives less compensatory demand. The exhale-on-lift technique also trains the pelvic floor to engage automatically during exertion, which is the coordination needed for leakage prevention during real-life effort.

> ### *Progression: Single-Leg Bridge*
> *Once you can perform three sets of ten bridges comfortably with good form, you are ready for the single-leg variation. From the top of a standard bridge, extend one leg straight out so it is parallel to the floor, keeping the hips level and not allowing one side to drop. Hold for two seconds, then return the foot to the mat and lower. Perform five repetitions on each side. This progression adds hip stabilizer demand and significantly increases the challenge to the pelvic floor and deep abdominals. Only attempt the single-leg variation after two to three weeks of consistent standard bridge practice.*

2. Clamshell

The clamshell targets the gluteus medius, the outer hip muscle most responsible for pelvic stability during walking and single-leg movements. Weakness here is one of the most common contributors to pelvic instability in women over 60.

Starting Position:

Lie on your right side on a firm mat with your hips and knees bent at approximately 45 degrees, your knees stacked on top of each other, and your feet together. Rest your head on your right arm or on a folded towel. Your hips are stacked vertically and your spine is in a straight line.

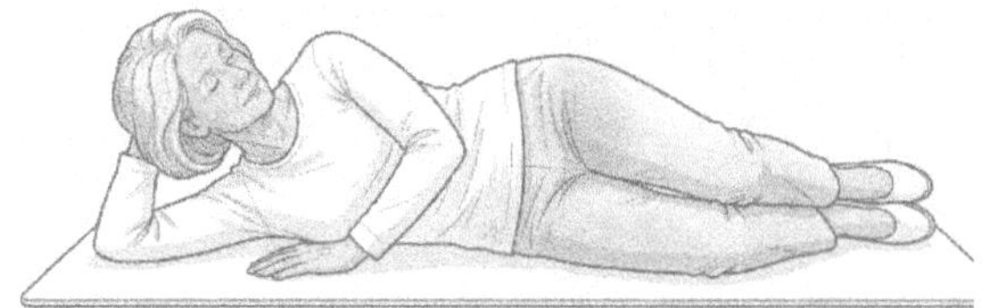

Steps:

1. Breathe in to prepare.

2. As you breathe out, keep your feet together and rotate your top knee upward, opening like a clamshell. Lift only as far as you can without your hips rolling backward.

3. Hold the lifted position for two seconds, feeling the work in the outer left hip.

4. Breathe in and lower the knee slowly back to the starting position.

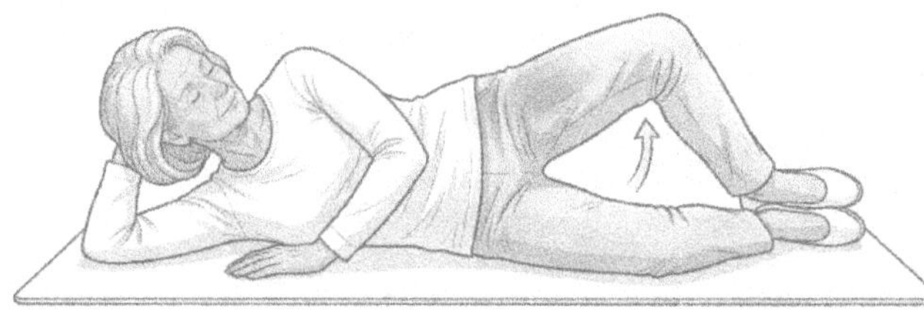

5. Repeat for the full set on the right side, then roll to your left side and repeat with the right leg lifting.

6. Each lift and lower counts as one repetition.

Reps / Hold: 12 repetitions each side
Sets: 3 sets each side

If this feels difficult: If rotating your hip causes discomfort, reduce the range of the lift significantly and focus on the sensation of engagement in the outer hip rather than the height of the movement. Even a small lift with correct muscle recruitment is effective.

Why this works: A strong gluteus medius keeps the pelvis level during every step you take. When this muscle is weak, the pelvis drops on the opposite side with each stride, which continuously destabilizes the pelvic floor. This exercise directly addresses the hip stability foundation that pelvic floor function depends on during daily movement.

3. Modified Bird-Dog

The modified bird-dog trains the deep abdominals and lower back stabilizers to maintain a neutral spine against opposing limb movement, which is exactly the demand placed on your core every time you reach, carry, or walk.

Starting Position:

Begin on your hands and knees on a firm mat, with your wrists directly below your shoulders and your knees directly below your hips. Your spine is in a neutral position, neither arched nor rounded. The back of your neck is long and your gaze is toward the mat.

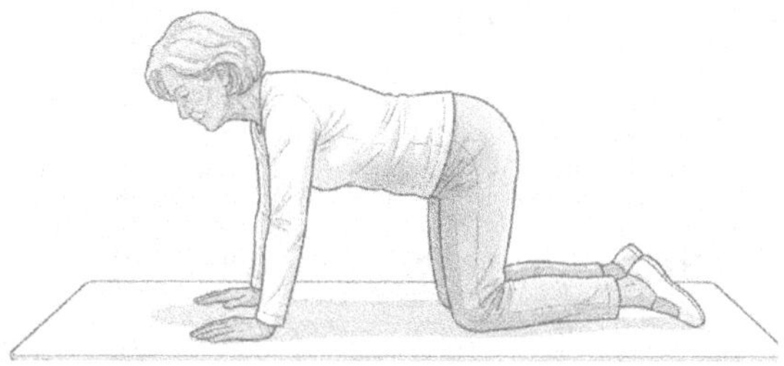

Steps:

1. Breathe in to prepare. Gently draw your lower belly upward without changing your spine position.

2. As you breathe out, slowly extend your right arm forward to shoulder height and your left leg back to hip height simultaneously.

3. Hold for three seconds. Your hips must remain level. Do not allow your lower back to arch or your hips to rotate.

4. Breathe in and slowly return your arm and leg to the starting position.

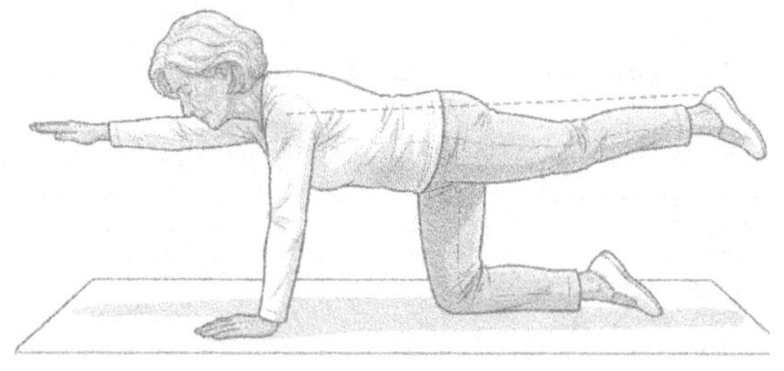

5. Repeat on the opposite side: left arm forward and right leg back. That is one full repetition.

6. Move slowly and with control. Speed is not the goal. Stillness during the hold is.

Reps / Hold: 8 repetitions each side
Sets: 3 sets

If this feels difficult: If getting onto hands and knees is uncomfortable for the wrists or knees, perform this exercise standing at a kitchen counter or sturdy table. Place both hands on the surface for support, hinge forward from the hips until your back is roughly parallel to the floor, and then lift one leg straight back to hip height. Hold for three seconds and lower. The spinal stability demand is identical to the floor version.

Why this works: The bird-dog directly trains the ability to maintain a stable, neutral pelvis while the limbs move, which is the core skill needed for walking, carrying, and reaching without pelvic floor pressure. The contralateral arm and leg pattern also engages the deep spinal stabilizers that work alongside the pelvic floor during rotation and balance.

4. Supported Squat

The supported squat builds the leg and glute strength needed for the most demanding functional movement of daily life: sitting down and standing up. Using a chair for support removes the balance challenge so the strength work remains the primary focus.

Starting Position:

Stand in front of a sturdy chair with your feet hip-width apart and toes pointing slightly outward. The chair is directly behind you. Rest your hands lightly on the back of a second chair or a kitchen counter placed in front of you for balance support.

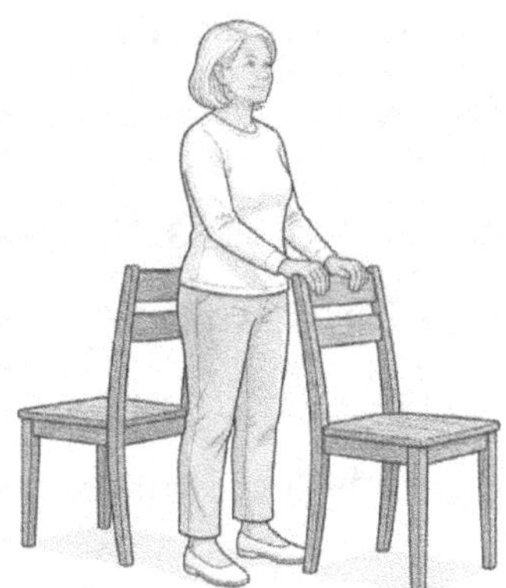

Steps:

1. Breathe in to prepare.

2. As you breathe out, push your hips backward and bend both knees, lowering your body as though you are about to sit down.

3. Lower until your thighs are approaching parallel to the floor or until you gently touch the chair seat behind you.

4. Pause for one second at the bottom, keeping your chest lifted and your knees tracking over your toes.

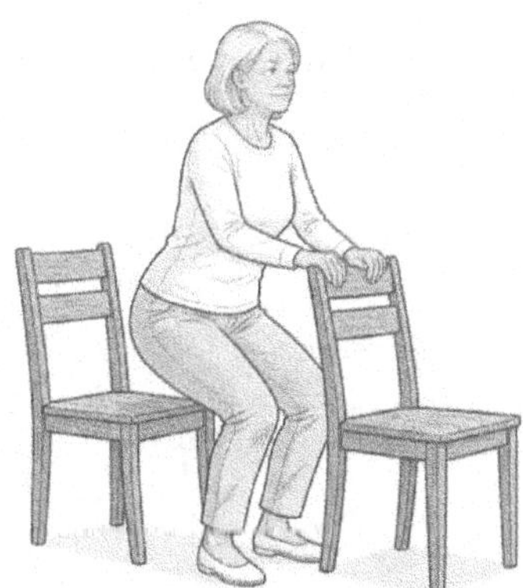

5. As you breathe in, press through both heels and straighten your legs to return to standing.

6. Squeeze your glutes gently as you reach full standing height.

Reps / Hold: 10 repetitions
Sets: 3 sets

If this feels difficult: If lowering to near parallel causes knee discomfort, reduce the depth to a quarter squat and focus on the sensation of pressing through the heels to rise.

Over several weeks, the range of motion typically increases as the surrounding muscles strengthen. Never lower into pain.

Why this works: Getting out of a chair is the single most demanding functional movement most women over 60 perform multiple times daily. Building strength in this exact pattern reduces the compensatory strain on the lower back and pelvic floor during every chair rise, while also improving the balance and confidence needed for stair climbing and uneven surfaces.

5. Standing Side Leg Raise

The standing side leg raise builds the outer hip and gluteus medius in a standing, weight-bearing position, which is closer to how these muscles actually function during walking than any floor-based alternative.

Starting Position:

Stand upright beside a wall, sturdy chair, or kitchen counter with your right hand resting lightly on the surface for balance. Both feet are hip-width apart, toes pointing forward. Stand tall with your weight evenly distributed and your core lightly engaged.

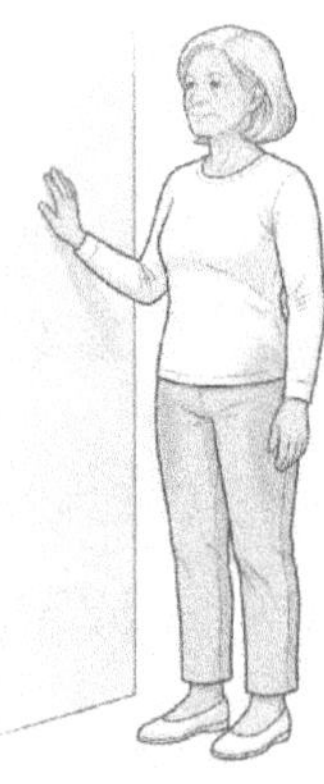

Steps:
1. Breathe in to prepare. Shift your weight gently onto your right foot, keeping the right knee soft, not locked.

2. As you breathe out, lift your left leg out to the side, keeping your toes pointing forward and your hip facing forward.

3. Lift to a height that is comfortable, typically 12 to 18 inches from the floor. Do not tilt your upper body to the side to compensate.

4. Hold for two seconds at the top of the lift.

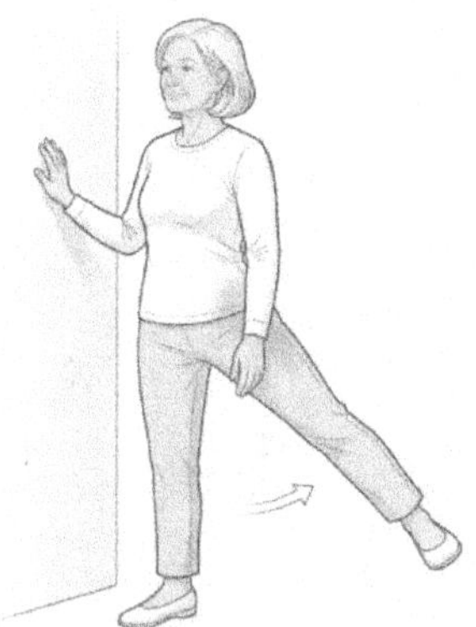

5. As you breathe in, slowly lower your left foot back to the floor.

6. Complete the full set on the left side, then switch hands and repeat with the right leg lifting.

Reps / Hold: 12 repetitions each side
Sets: 3 sets each side

If this feels difficult: If maintaining balance on one foot feels unstable, place both hands on the wall or counter rather than one. Stability and confidence take priority over independence from the support surface. As balance improves over the first two to three weeks, gradually reduce the hand contact until you are using just one or two fingertips.

Why this works: Walking is a continuous series of single-leg balance moments. The gluteus medius must fire strongly to keep the pelvis level during each stride. When it does not, the pelvis drops and shifts, creating a downward pressure load on the pelvic floor with every step. This exercise trains the standing hip stability that reduces that repetitive daily load.

6. Wall Sit with Core Activation

The wall sit builds isometric quad and glute endurance while the core activation layer trains the deep abdominals and pelvic floor to hold their coordinated engagement under sustained load, which is the exact demand of prolonged standing and walking.

Starting Position:

Stand with your back flat against a smooth, sturdy wall. Your feet are hip-width apart and positioned about 18 inches in front of the wall. Your arms rest at your sides or across your chest.

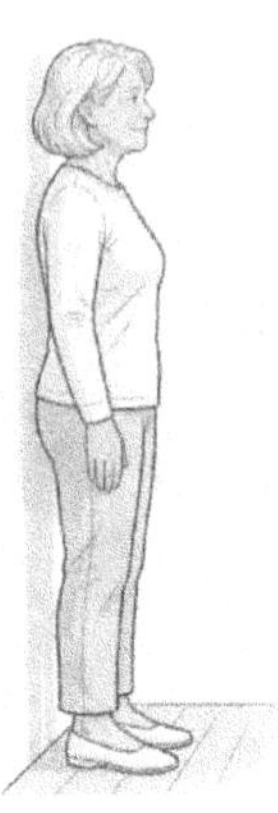

Steps:

1. Breathe in and lengthen your spine against the wall.

2. As you breathe out, slide your back down the wall, bending both knees until your thighs are at approximately 45 degrees. Do not go to full parallel if this causes knee discomfort.

3. Press your lower back firmly against the wall and gently draw your lower belly inward to engage your deep abdominals.

4. Hold this position and breathe slowly and normally. Add a gentle pelvic floor lift on each exhale if possible.

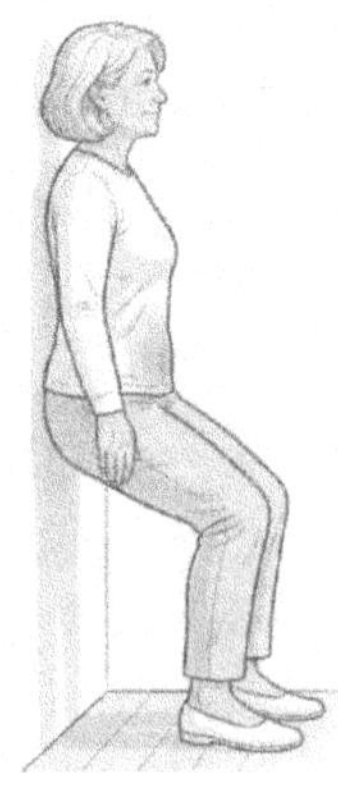

5. Hold for the target duration, maintaining normal breathing and the light abdominal engagement throughout.

6. To come out, press through both heels and slide back up the wall to standing.

Reps / Hold: Hold for 20 to 30 seconds. Build toward 45 seconds over 4 weeks.
Sets: 3 sets, with 60-second rest between sets

If this feels difficult: If 45 degrees causes knee discomfort, raise the angle so your knees bend only slightly. Even a 20-degree bend against the wall with active core engagement provides meaningful strength and endurance training. Reduce the hold time as well if needed, beginning with 10-second holds and building week by week.

Why this works: Sustained postural muscle endurance is what determines whether your core continues to support your pelvic floor during the eighth hour of a day, not just the first. This exercise builds the slow-twitch muscle endurance in the quadriceps, glutes, and deep abdominals that translates directly into reduced pelvic floor fatigue during prolonged standing and activity.

Chapter 7

Bladder Control Exercises — Regaining Control

This is the chapter most women came for. The one they flipped to first before reading anything else. That makes sense, and there is no judgment in saying it: if leakage or urgency is the thing that brought you to this book, then this is where the most direct work begins.

These five exercises address the symptoms you are living with every day. They are practical, specific, and written for the moments when the problem actually shows up, not just for practice sessions on a mat.

There are two distinct patterns of bladder control difficulty, and they respond to different exercises. Stress incontinence is leakage caused by sudden physical pressure: a cough, a sneeze, a laugh, getting up quickly, or lifting something. The pelvic floor muscles fail to close fast enough against the spike in abdominal pressure. Exercises 1 and 3 in this chapter address this pattern directly. Urgency incontinence is the sudden overwhelming need to reach the bathroom, sometimes accompanied by leakage before arrival. The bladder contracts without permission, and no amount of squeezing seems to stop it. Exercises 2, 4, and 5 address urgency. Many women experience both patterns at different times. Working through all five exercises in sequence addresses both.

Bladder Control Exercises

1. Quick-Flick Kegels

The Quick-Flick Kegel trains the fast-twitch pelvic floor muscle fibers that are responsible for the rapid reflex closure needed when a sneeze or cough arrives. This is the exercise that directly addresses stress leakage during sudden pressure events.

Think of the moment just before a sneeze when you feel it building. That two-second window is where the Quick-Flick Kegel operates. Training this fast contraction in practice sessions builds the reflex speed that eventually fires automatically in real life, even before you consciously register the sneeze coming.

Starting Position:

Sit upright on a firm chair with both feet flat on the floor, hip-width apart, and your hands resting on your thighs. Your spine is tall and your jaw and shoulders are relaxed.

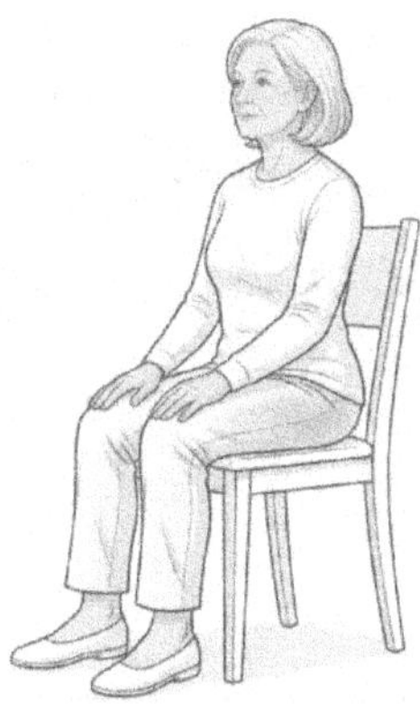

Steps:

1. Breathe in slowly and let your pelvic floor fully relax.

2. As you breathe out, perform a fast, sharp pelvic floor contraction and release it immediately. The hold lasts only one second.

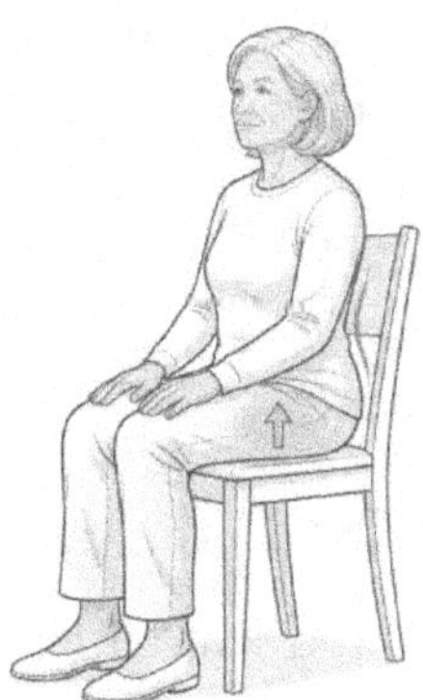

3. Rest for two seconds, then repeat: contract sharply, release immediately.

4. Continue the quick contract-and-release pattern at a steady rhythm.

5. After completing the set, breathe slowly for 30 seconds before the next set.

6. Focus on the sharpness of the contraction rather than the strength. Speed is the training goal here.

Reps / Hold: 10 quick contractions per set
Sets: 3 sets, with 30-second rest between sets

If this feels difficult: If quick contractions feel impossible to isolate from other muscles, begin with slow Kegels from Chapter 5 for one week to establish the muscle connection, then introduce the quick-flick pattern once you can reliably contract without recruiting your thighs or buttocks.

Why this works: Stress leakage happens when the pelvic floor fast-twitch fibers do not fire quickly enough to close the urethra before abdominal pressure arrives. These quick-flick repetitions directly train that speed of response, building the reflex needed to stay dry during coughing, sneezing, and physical effort.

2. Endurance Holds

Endurance Holds build the slow-twitch pelvic floor muscle fibers responsible for sustained closure during prolonged standing, walking, and the accumulation of activity across a full day. This exercise addresses the leakage pattern that tends to appear later in the day when the muscles have fatigued.

Many women notice their symptoms are worse in the afternoon or evening than in the morning. This is not a coincidence. The slow-twitch fibers that maintain baseline pelvic floor tone throughout the day fatigue just like any postural muscle. Endurance Holds train these fibers to sustain their function for longer before they tire.

Starting Position:

Sit upright on a firm chair with both feet flat on the floor, hip-width apart. Rest your hands on your thighs and establish normal relaxed breathing before you begin.

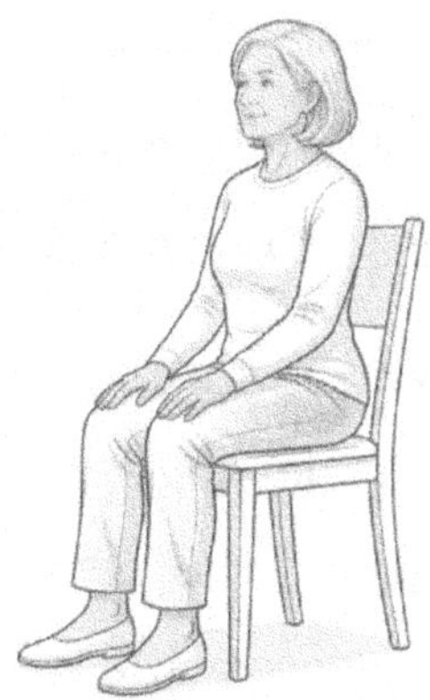

Steps:

1. Breathe in and allow your pelvic floor to fully relax.

2. As you breathe out, gently lift and squeeze the pelvic floor muscles to about 50 percent of your maximum effort. This is a moderate, sustained hold, not your hardest contraction.

3. Hold the contraction and continue breathing normally throughout. Do not hold your breath.

4. Count the hold time slowly in your head. Work toward the target hold time without straining.

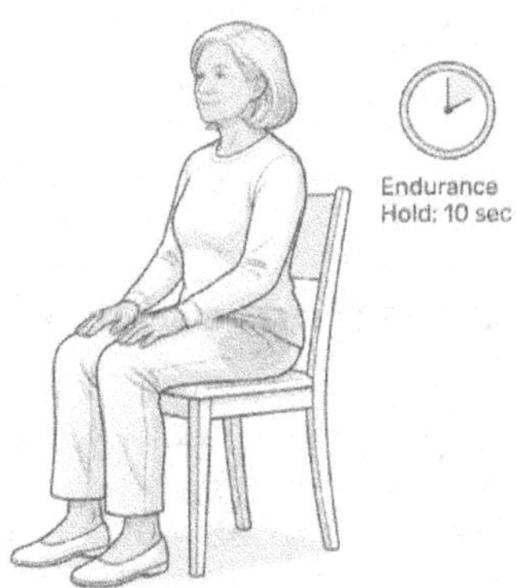

5. When the hold time is reached, release slowly and completely over five seconds.

6. Rest for 10 seconds before the next hold. The rest is not optional: the slow-twitch fibers need recovery time to adapt.

Reps / Hold: Begin with 8-second holds. Build to 10 seconds by Week 3, then 12 seconds by Week 4.

Sets: 8 to 10 holds per set, 3 sets

If this feels difficult: If holding for 8 seconds causes you to recruit your buttocks or hold your breath, shorten the hold to 4 seconds and build gradually. A 4-second hold with correct muscle isolation is more effective than an 8-second hold using the wrong muscles.

Why this works: The slow-twitch pelvic floor fibers maintain continuous low-level tone throughout the day. When they fatigue, leakage appears. Training endurance holds specifically develops these fibers, extending the period of sustained protection during prolonged standing, walking, and activity across the full day.

3. Functional Kegel

The Functional Kegel bridges the gap between practice sessions and real life. It is a protocol for deliberately applying a pelvic floor contraction at the specific moments in daily life when leakage is most likely to occur. The goal is to make the contraction an automatic habit rather than a reactive scramble.

How the Functional Kegel Works:

Before any movement or event that typically causes leakage, you perform one deliberate pelvic floor contraction and hold it through the event. The contraction is maintained from the moment before the pressure arrives until the pressure has fully passed. Over weeks of consistent practice, this timed contraction begins to happen automatically without conscious effort.

Application Moment 1: Standing from a Chair

Before you begin to push yourself up from a seated position, exhale and gently contract your pelvic floor. Maintain the contraction as you rise to full standing height. Hold until you are fully upright and steady, then release. Getting out of a chair is one of the highest-pressure moments for the pelvic floor, and applying the contraction before the effort begins rather than after leakage starts is the key difference this exercise trains.

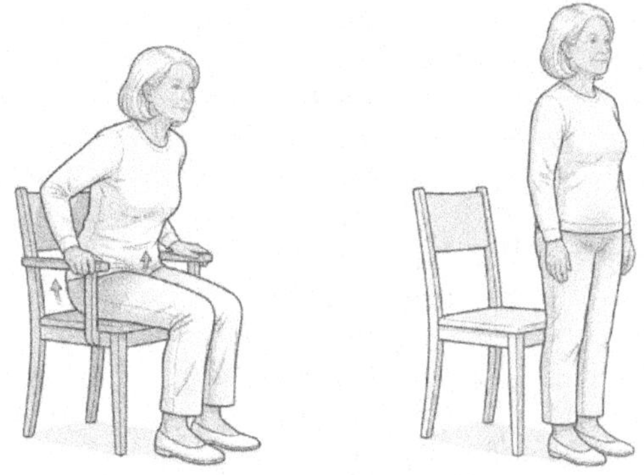

Engage (Left Panel) and Maintain (Right Panel)

Application Moment 2: Picking Something Up

Before you bend forward to pick up an object from a low surface, exhale and contract. Keep the contraction in place as you bend, grasp the object, and return to standing. Release after you are fully upright. Bending forward creates a forward pressure wave in the abdomen that arrives at the pelvic floor faster than an unprepared muscle can respond. The pre-contraction intercepts that pressure at the source.

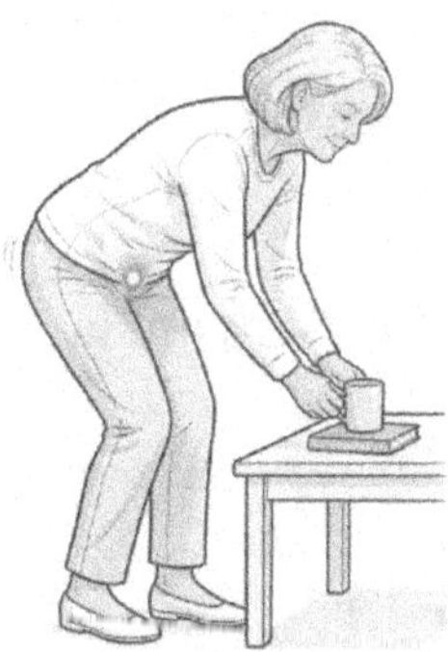

Application Moment 3: A Sudden Laugh

This one is less controllable than the other two because laughter arrives without warning. The goal is not to suppress laughter but to train the reflex speed so the pelvic floor contracts reflexively when you feel laughter starting. The Quick-Flick Kegels in Exercise 1 build this reflex speed. The Functional Kegel practice gives you the conscious repetition that eventually becomes unconscious. When you feel laughter beginning, contract sharply and hold until the laughter settles. Over weeks, this sequence shortens until the contraction arrives before you have consciously initiated it.

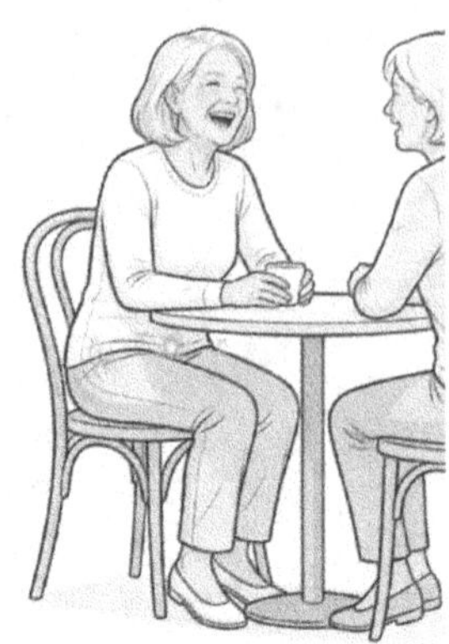

Reps / Hold: Practice each application moment deliberately at least 5 times per day
Sets: Ongoing daily practice, not a structured set sequence

If this feels difficult: If applying the contraction before the moment consistently proves difficult, start with just one application moment: chair rises only. Practice this exclusively for the first week until the sequence becomes habitual, then add the bending application in Week 2, and the laugh application as awareness builds.

Why this works: Stress leakage is a timing problem. The pelvic floor contraction arrives after the pressure event rather than before it. The Functional Kegel trains the timing so the contraction precedes the pressure, which is the only position from which it can successfully prevent leakage. This exercise translates every minute of mat-based practice into a real-life result.

4. Urge Suppression Technique

The Urge Suppression Technique is a step-by-step in-the-moment protocol for managing sudden bladder urgency without rushing to the bathroom. It works by using the pelvic floor and nervous system to override the bladder contraction signal before it escalates into leakage.

Urgency feels uncontrollable because the bladder muscle contracts involuntarily and sends an urgent signal to the brain. But the signal is not always accurate. The bladder contracts long before it is actually full, creating urgency out of habit rather than genuine need. The protocol below interrupts that habitual signal pattern and teaches the bladder that the urgent feeling does not require immediate action.

The In-the-Moment Urge Suppression Protocol:

1. When urgency strikes, stop moving. Stand still or sit down if possible.

2. Take a slow, deep breath in through your nose. Do not rush toward the bathroom.

3. Perform three to five Quick-Flick Kegels in rapid succession. This signals the bladder to relax.

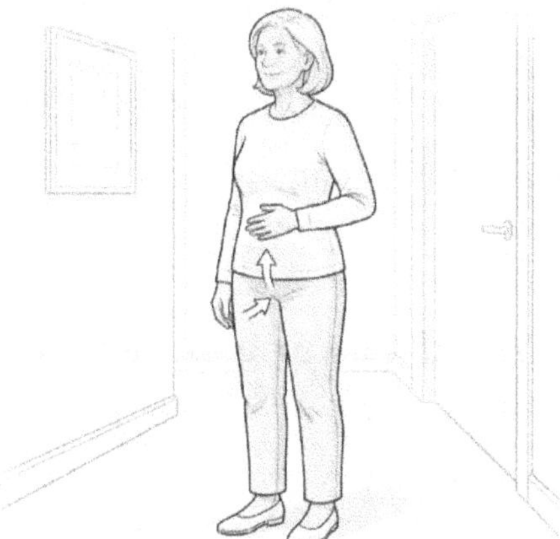

4. Take another slow breath out. Let your shoulders and abdomen relax completely.

5. Wait for 60 to 90 seconds. The urgency should begin to subside. If it does not, perform three more Quick-Flicks.

6. Once the urgency has reduced, walk calmly to the bathroom. Do not run.

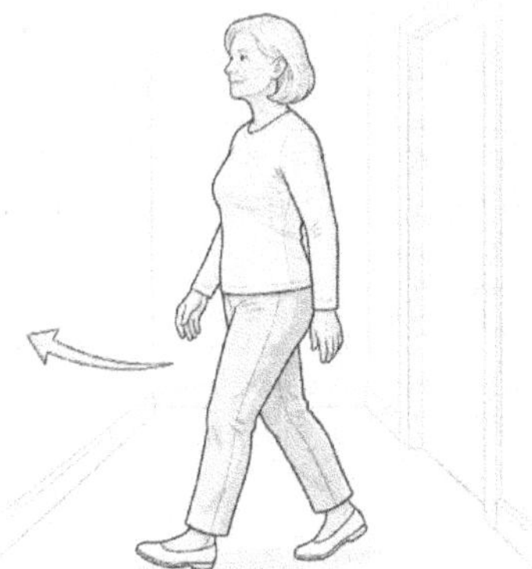

Reps / Hold: Practice the protocol every time urgency occurs throughout the day
Sets: Ongoing daily practice

If this feels difficult: If the urge arrives suddenly while you are moving, prioritize stopping first. Standing still is the single most effective first step because walking and especially running increase abdominal pressure and worsen urgency. If stopping is not possible, slow your pace significantly and focus on the breathing and Quick-Flick sequence while continuing to move slowly.

Why this works: The pelvic floor has a direct neurological connection to the bladder. When pelvic floor muscles contract, they send an inhibitory signal to the bladder muscle that reduces its urgency contraction. This technique uses that reflex deliberately and consistently to retrain the bladder away from its habitual overactivity pattern.

The timed voiding schedule below works alongside the Urge Suppression Technique to gradually extend the time between bathroom visits, rebuilding the bladder's capacity over seven days.

Urge Suppression: 7-Day Timed Voiding Schedule

Day	Target Interval	Goal	Notes
Day 1	45 to 60 minutes	Do not rush to bathroom on first urge	Log any leakage. Note what triggered the urge.
Day 2	60 minutes	Use the protocol before walking to bathroom	Focus on the stop-and-breathe step first.
Day 3	60 to 75 minutes	Wait 5 minutes after urge before going	Urgency should feel more manageable by now.
Day 4	75 minutes	Consistently wait before going	Some days will be harder than others. Stay consistent.
Day 5	75 to 90 minutes	Wait 10 minutes after urge before going	Increase fluid intake slightly if reducing it was a habit.
Day 6	90 minutes	Begin combining with bladder retraining	If urgency is well-controlled, extend intervals further.
Day 7	90 to 105 minutes	Approach 2-hour intervals comfortably	Consult healthcare provider if no improvement has occurred.

5. Bladder Retraining Protocol

The Bladder Retraining Protocol is a structured approach to gradually extending the time between bathroom visits over seven days. It works by combining the Urge Suppression

Technique with a deliberate schedule, progressively lengthening the bladder's functional capacity and reducing the frequency and unpredictability of urgency.

Many women with urgency have inadvertently trained their bladder to signal early and often by visiting the bathroom at the first hint of urge rather than waiting. The bladder learns this pattern and begins contracting earlier and earlier. Retraining reverses that pattern by introducing controlled delay, allowing the bladder to stretch gently back toward a more functional capacity.

Starting Position:

This protocol is practiced throughout your waking day, not during a specific exercise session. Begin it on a day when you will be at home and able to monitor your bathroom visits without the pressure of commitments or travel.

How to Follow the Protocol:

1. Record the time of your first bathroom visit of the morning. This is your starting point.

2. Set a target interval from the table below. Do not go to the bathroom before that time has elapsed unless leakage is imminent.

3. When urgency arrives before your interval is complete, use the Urge Suppression Technique from Exercise 4.

4. When your interval time arrives, go to the bathroom whether you feel a strong urge or not.

5. Record each visit, any leakage episodes, and how intense the urgency felt on a scale of 1 to 5.

6. Each day, extend the interval slightly. Follow the 7-day schedule below as your guide.

7. Do not reduce fluid intake as a strategy. Concentrated urine irritates the bladder lining and worsens urgency. Aim for six to eight glasses of water across the day.

Reps / Hold: Follow the schedule throughout the full waking day, every day for 7 days
Sets: Ongoing daily protocol

If this feels difficult: If extending intervals causes significant distress or repeated leakage on the first day, begin with a shorter baseline interval of 30 minutes and build from there. Progress is individual. Some women reach 90-minute intervals by Day 7 and others take two to three weeks. Both are normal outcomes.

Why this works: Bladder urgency is largely a learned pattern. The bladder can be retrained through consistent, graduated delay because the urge signal is managed by the brain as much as by the bladder itself. Structured retraining reduces the frequency of urgency episodes, extends functional bladder capacity, and breaks the cycle of anticipatory bathroom visits that reinforce the overactive pattern.

Bladder Retraining: 7-Day Interval Schedule

Day	Target Interval	Urgency Management	Notes
Day 1	Your current average	Use urge suppression at every urge	Do not restrict fluids. Log all visits and urgency rating.
Day 2	Add 10 minutes	Use urge suppression at every urge	Small increase only. Do not jump ahead.
Day 3	Add 10 more minutes	Protocol becoming more familiar	If leakage increases, hold Day 2 interval for another day.
Day 4	Hold the new interval	Focus on maintaining consistency	Consistency builds the new pattern. Do not skip.
Day 5	Add 10 more minutes	Urge should be less intense by now	Increase fluid to 7 or 8 glasses if not already there.
Day 6	Hold the new interval	Consolidate and maintain	Use the Urge Suppression protocol every single time.
Day 7	Add 10 more minutes	Note final comfortable interval	Continue weekly at this interval before increasing further.

Chapter 8

Mobility Exercises — Moving Freely with Confidence

Moving freely is the third promise in the subtitle of this book, and it is the one that is easiest to overlook when bladder control is the most pressing concern. But the two are not separate goals. The hip flexibility, spinal mobility, and inner thigh release trained in this chapter directly reduce the structural tension that loads the pelvic floor from the outside.

Tight hip flexors tilt the pelvis forward and pull on the pelvic floor attachment points, placing the muscles in a chronically lengthened, weakened position before any exercise even begins. A stiff lower back limits the thoracic mobility needed for correct diaphragmatic breathing, disrupting the pressure rhythm that the pelvic floor depends on. Restricted inner thigh muscles brace the entire inner pelvic region, creating a holding pattern that keeps the pelvic floor in a state of low-level chronic tension. Every exercise in this chapter addresses one of these structural contributors. Each "Why this works" note connects specifically to what that restriction costs the pelvic floor, not just what it costs your general flexibility.

Mobility Exercises

1. Hip Flexor Stretch

This stretch targets the iliopsoas, the deep hip flexor that runs from the lumbar spine through the pelvis to the inner thigh. Chronic shortening of this muscle is among the most common structural contributors to pelvic floor dysfunction in women who spend extended periods sitting each day.

Starting Position:

Stand beside a sturdy chair, placing your right hand on the back of the chair for balance. Step your right foot forward and your left foot back, creating a wide split stance. Both feet point forward. Your front knee remains above your front ankle.

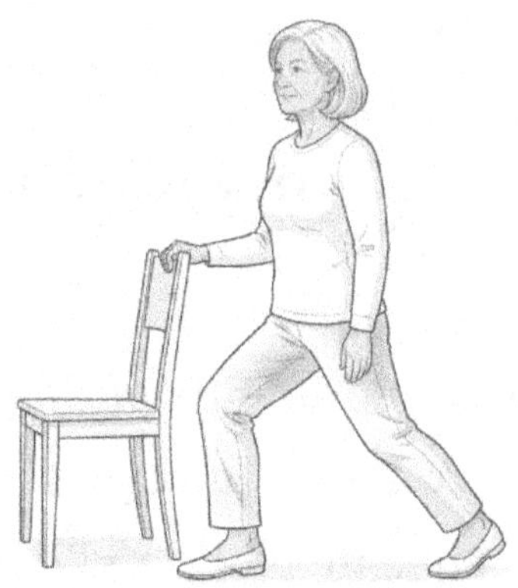

Steps:

1. Breathe in to prepare and lengthen your spine upward.

2. As you breathe out, gently bend your front knee forward, shifting your weight toward the front foot.

3. Keep your back heel on the floor and your back leg straight. Feel the stretch in the front of your left hip and thigh.

4. Hold the stretch and breathe slowly and fully into the sensation. Do not lean your upper body forward.

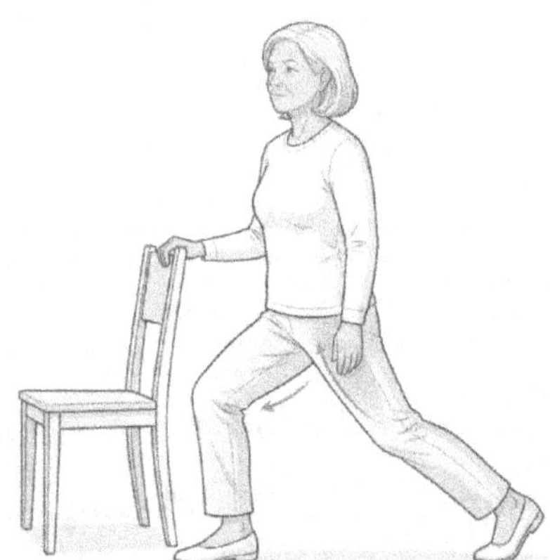

5. After holding, breathe in and gently straighten your front knee to return to the starting stance.

6. Switch sides, placing your left foot forward and right foot back, and repeat the full sequence.

Reps / Hold: Hold for 25 to 30 seconds each side
Sets: 2 sets each side

If this feels difficult: If the full split stance causes balance difficulty, perform this stretch at a kitchen counter with both hands resting on the surface. Alternatively, reduce the length of the stance so the weight shift is smaller and the stretch intensity is gentler.

Why this works: The iliopsoas attaches directly to the lumbar vertebrae and runs through the pelvis, putting it in direct anatomical contact with the pelvic floor's attachment zone. A shortened iliopsoas tilts the pelvis anteriorly and compresses the lumbar spine, pulling the pelvic floor into a chronically overstretched position that reduces its strength and responsiveness. Releasing this muscle restores the neutral pelvic alignment in which the pelvic floor can generate its best force output.

2. Inner Thigh Release

The inner thigh muscles, specifically the adductors, share fascial connections and neurological pathways with the pelvic floor. Inner thigh tension and pelvic floor tension frequently travel together: releasing one consistently reduces the other, making this stretch one of the most direct access points for reducing pelvic floor overactivity from the outside.

Starting Position:

Sit on the floor or on a firm mat with your back resting against a wall for support. Bring the soles of your feet together in front of you and let your knees drop outward toward the floor. Rest your hands on your feet or your ankles.

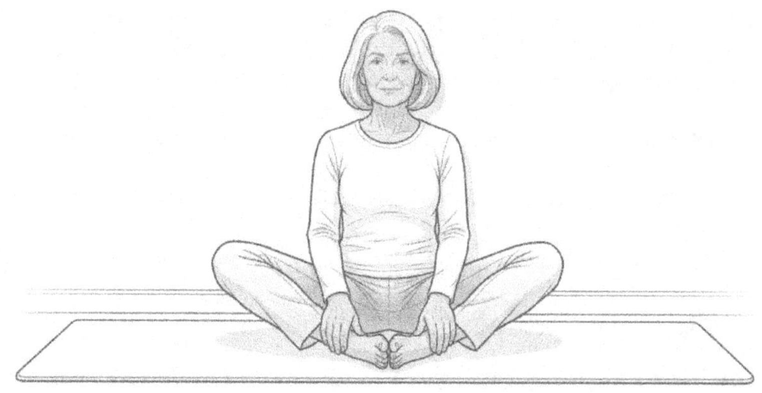

Steps:

1. Breathe in slowly and sit as tall as possible against the wall.

2. As you breathe out, gently allow your knees to drop a little further toward the floor. Do not press them down with your hands.

3. Hold the position and breathe slowly. On each exhale, consciously release any inner thigh gripping and allow gravity to deepen the stretch.

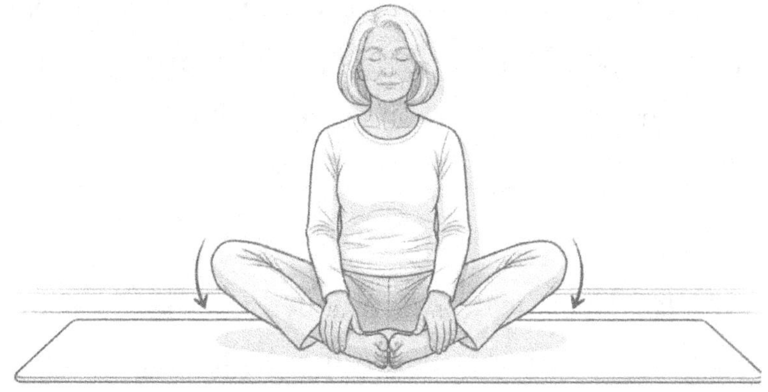

4. Add a pelvic floor release on each inhale: as you breathe in, allow both the inner thighs and the pelvic floor to soften simultaneously.

5. Maintain the hold, continuing to breathe slowly and release on each exhale.

6. To come out, use your hands to gently bring your knees back upward before slowly extending your legs.

Reps / Hold: Hold for 30 to 45 seconds
Sets: 2 sets

If this feels difficult: If sitting on the floor is uncomfortable, perform this stretch seated on a firm chair. Cross one ankle over the opposite knee in a figure-four position and allow the crossed knee to drop outward gently. This delivers a similar inner thigh and external hip rotator release from a seated position without requiring floor work.

Why this works: The adductors and the pelvic floor share fascia along the inner pelvic ring. When the adductors are chronically tight, they create inward compressive force on the pelvic floor from both sides, sustaining a background level of tension that prevents the pelvic floor from fully releasing between contractions. Releasing inner thigh tension directly reduces this background load, which is particularly beneficial for women with overactivity, urgency, or pelvic discomfort.

3. Lower Back Mobility Roll

The Lower Back Mobility Roll decompresses the lumbar spine and sacrum and restores the gentle rocking mobility of the pelvis that stiffens with prolonged sitting. This movement directly releases the lower back tension that limits pelvic floor range of motion.

Starting Position:

Lie on your back on a firm mat with your knees bent and your feet flat on the floor, hip-width apart. Rest your arms at your sides with palms facing down. Take two slow breaths and allow your body to relax into the mat before beginning.

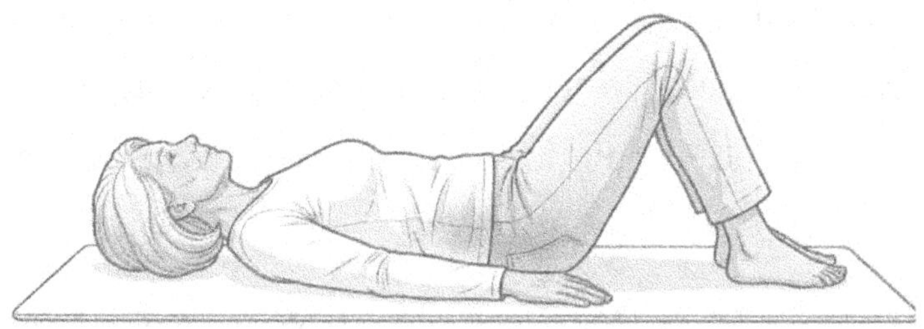

Steps:
1. Breathe in slowly and allow your lower back to find its neutral arch.

2. As you breathe out, tilt your pelvis gently backward, pressing your lower back toward the mat.

3. As you breathe in, tilt your pelvis forward, allowing your lower back to arch slightly away from the mat.

4. Continue rocking slowly between these two positions in time with your breath, creating a gentle rolling motion through the lower back.

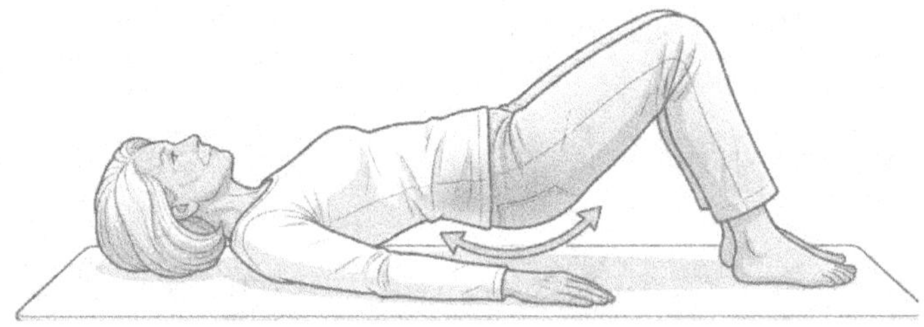

5. After the gentle rolls, draw both knees toward your chest and hold briefly to release the lower back fully.

6. Slowly extend both legs back to flat and rest for three breaths before completing the second set.

Reps / Hold: 10 full rock cycles, synchronized with breath
Sets: 2 sets

If this feels difficult: If tilting the pelvis causes lower back discomfort, reduce the range of movement to a very small rock. Even a slight shift between neutral and minimally tilted delivers the joint mobility and circulation benefits without requiring a large movement range.

Why this works: The sacrum is the posterior attachment point for several pelvic floor muscle groups. When the lower back and sacroiliac joints are stiff, they limit the sacrum's natural micro-movement, which in turn restricts the pelvic floor's full range of motion during breathing and exercise. Restoring this gentle lower back mobility frees the sacrum to move as designed, directly expanding the pelvic floor's available range and responsiveness.

4. Cat-Cow with Pelvic Floor Coordination

Cat-Cow coordinates spinal flexion and extension with breathing and deliberate pelvic floor movement, making it the most complete integration exercise in this chapter. The three-position sequence trains the full pelvic floor range: release on inhalation and extension, gentle lift on exhalation and flexion.

Starting Position — Neutral Spine:

Begin on your hands and knees on a firm mat, with your wrists directly below your shoulders and your knees directly below your hips. Your spine is in a neutral position, neither arched nor rounded, forming a flat tabletop from the base of the skull to the tailbone.

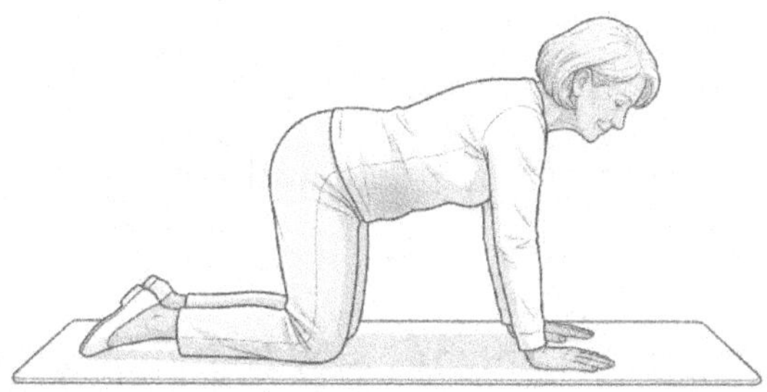

Steps — Cat Position:

1. As you breathe out, draw your lower belly gently upward, round your spine toward the ceiling, and tuck your tailbone down and under.

2. Let your head drop gently downward as your spine rounds. Hold for two seconds.

3. During the cat position, allow the pelvic floor to gently lift with the exhale and the spinal flexion.

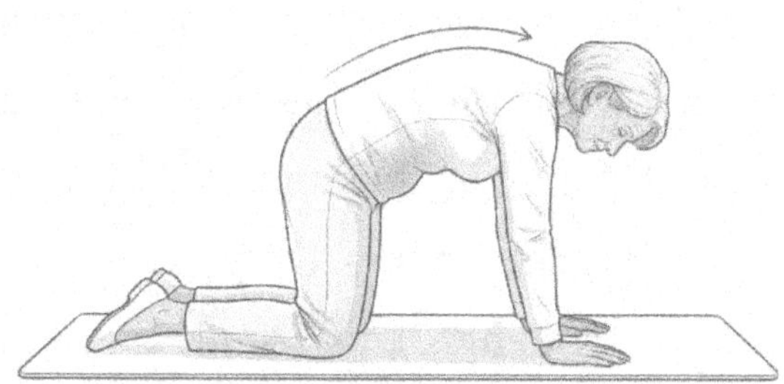

Steps — Cow Position:

4. As you breathe in, let your belly drop toward the mat, allow your lower back to gently arch, and lift your tailbone upward.

5. Lift your gaze forward slightly as your spine extends into the cow position. Hold for two seconds.

6. During the cow position, allow the pelvic floor to soften and gently drop with the inhale and the spinal extension.

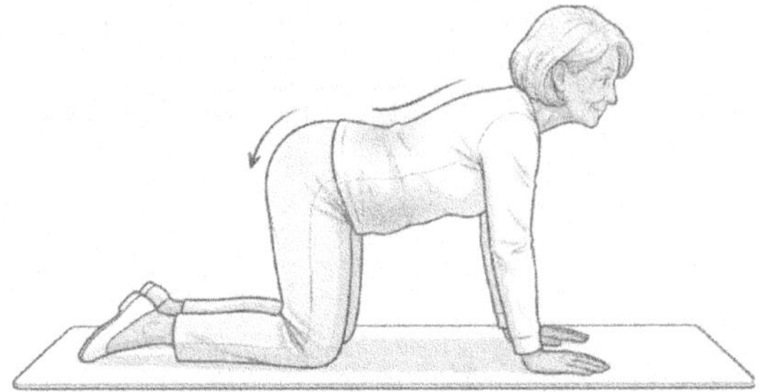

7. Return to neutral spine between each cat and cow cycle. Do not rush through the transition.

Reps / Hold: 8 full cat-cow cycles, moving slowly and breathing with each position
Sets: 2 sets

If this feels difficult: If being on hands and knees causes wrist discomfort, make fists and rest on the flat of the knuckles rather than the open palm, which keeps the wrist in a neutral rather than extended position. Alternatively, rest on fists or use yoga blocks to reduce wrist extension. If knee discomfort is the issue, place a folded blanket under both knees before beginning.

Why this works: Cat-Cow trains the pelvic floor to move in coordination with spinal position and breath, which is the three-way integration that the exercises in Chapters 5 and 6 are built on. The pelvic floor naturally wants to lift on exhalation and spinal flexion, and release on inhalation and spinal extension. When this coordination pattern is disrupted by postural habits or muscle stiffness, the pelvic floor loses its timing advantage during exercise and daily movement. This sequence restores that coordination deliberately and progressively.

5. Seated Figure-Four Stretch

The Seated Figure-Four Stretch targets the piriformis and the deep hip external rotators, which lie directly adjacent to the pelvic floor and are among the most consistent sites of tension in women who carry pelvic floor overactivity.

Starting Position:

Sit upright on a firm chair with both feet flat on the floor, hip-width apart. Sit tall with your spine lengthened and your hands resting lightly on your thighs.

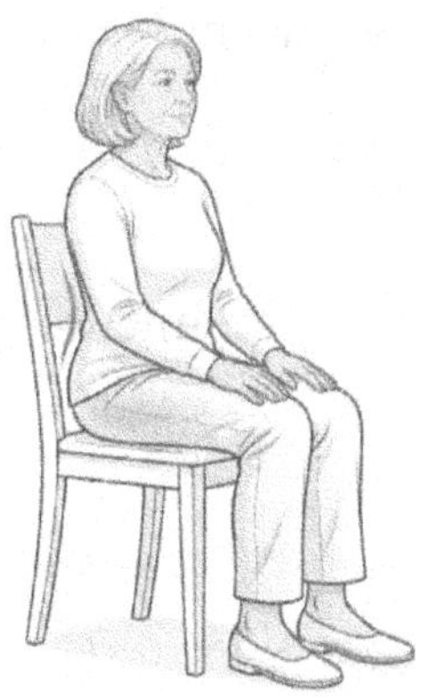

Steps:

1. Lift your right foot and cross it over your left knee, placing your right ankle just above the left kneecap.

2. Gently flex your right foot by drawing the toes back toward your shin. This protects the knee joint.

3. Sit tall. Feel the stretch in the outer right hip and gluteal area. If this is sufficient, stay here.

4. To deepen, breathe in to lengthen your spine, then as you breathe out, hinge gently forward from your hips.

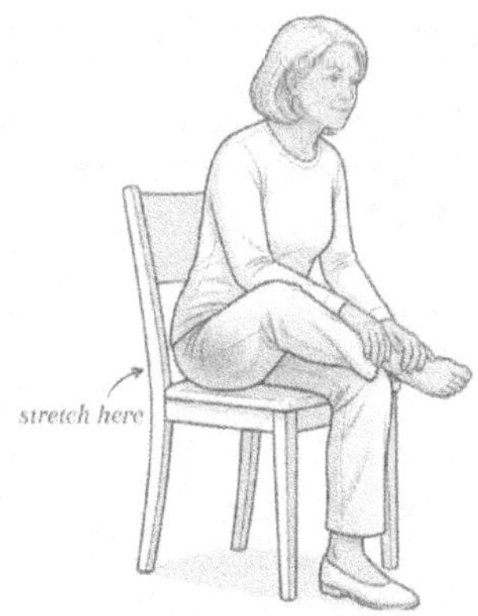

5. Hold the position, breathing slowly. Allow the outer hip to soften and release with each exhale.

6. Return to center, lower your right foot back to the floor, and repeat on the left side.

Reps / Hold: Hold for 25 to 30 seconds each side
Sets: 2 sets each side

If this feels difficult: If crossing your ankle over your knee is uncomfortable, move the ankle slightly lower toward the mid-shin rather than above the kneecap, which reduces the rotational demand on the hip joint. Alternatively, slide your right foot diagonally outward along the floor about 12 inches while keeping the heel down, creating a smaller external rotation that still accesses the target muscles.

Why this works: The piriformis and the obturator internus muscles share a direct fascial connection with the pelvic floor's lateral and posterior walls. When these muscles hold chronic tension, they pull on the pelvic floor from the outside, contributing to the overactive pattern that drives urgency, incomplete emptying, and pelvic discomfort. Stretching them consistently after every exercise session reduces this external load and helps the pelvic floor maintain the resting length needed for coordinated function during the exercises in Chapters 5 through 7.

Part IV: Your 4-Week Program And Beyond

Chapter 9

The 4-Week Illustrated Workout Program

A list of exercises is not a program. A program is a sequence, a progression, and a structure that builds on itself deliberately so that what you do in Week 1 makes Week 2 possible, and what you accomplish in Week 2 makes Week 3 more effective than it would have been if you had started there. That is exactly what this chapter provides.

How the Program Works

Each session in this program takes between 15 and 20 minutes. That is the full commitment: two to three minutes of warm-up, ten to twelve minutes of the main exercises, and three to five minutes of cool-down. Nothing here requires an hour. The sessions are short by design, because short sessions completed consistently produce better results than long sessions done occasionally.

The four weeks are built as a progressive sequence. Week 1 focuses exclusively on the foundation exercises and breathing from Chapter 5. The goal is not to tire the body. It is to establish the correct muscle patterns: diaphragmatic breathing, pelvic floor awareness, neutral pelvis, and deep abdominal engagement. These patterns are the scaffolding that every subsequent week is built on. Rushing past Week 1 because it feels easy undermines the coordination work that Week 2 depends on.

Week 2 introduces the core strength exercises from Chapter 6 alongside the foundations. The volume increases moderately and sessions become more demanding, but the breathing and pelvic floor coordination from Week 1 should now feel more automatic. Week 3 adds the bladder control exercises from Chapter 7 and increases the total sets across each session. By this point, most women notice that pelvic floor engagement feels more reliable and that symptoms have begun to shift. Week 4 integrates the mobility exercises from Chapter 8, raises endurance demands, and consolidates everything learned into a complete daily session.

If you miss a day, do not double up the following day. Return to the schedule and continue from where you left off. Missing one session does not reset your progress. Missing several in a row is best addressed by returning to the beginning of the current week rather than picking up mid-week.

Difficult weeks happen. Illness, travel, a poor night's sleep, or a flare of symptoms can make the standard session feel like too much. On those days, reduce the session to the three warm-up exercises, one set of Basic Kegels, and the Pelvic Floor Release Stretch. That is a complete session by any reasonable measure, and keeping the habit in place across difficult weeks matters more than maintaining full volume.

Progress in Week 1 is rarely dramatic. The early improvements are neurological: the brain is learning to locate and recruit the muscles more reliably. By Week 2, most women report a clearer sense of muscle engagement. By Week 3, functional improvements typically appear: less urgency, faster response to sudden pressure, improved daily awareness. By the end of Week 4, the program has become a habit with its own momentum. The goal from that point is to maintain and build on it.

Week 1 — Awareness

Week 1 is about finding the muscles, not fatiguing them. Every exercise this week comes from Chapter 4 warm-ups and Chapter 5 foundations. Sessions are gentle, deliberate, and focused on the three essentials: diaphragmatic breathing, pelvic floor awareness, and neutral pelvis alignment. Some days the muscle connection will feel clear; other days it will feel harder to locate. That is completely normal in the first week. Consistency is the only requirement. By Day 7, most women report a noticeably clearer sense of where the pelvic floor muscles are and what engaging them actually feels like.

Day	Exercises	Sets / Reps	Chapter Reference
Day 1	Seated Ankle Circles, Seated Knee Lifts, Shoulder Rolls | Basic Kegel, Pelvic Tilt, Diaphragmatic Breathing with Movement | Seated Forward Fold, Pelvic Floor Release	2 sets / 10 reps each	Ch. 4 warm-up | Ch. 5 | Ch. 4 cool-down
Day 2	REST DAY — Light walking encouraged	—	—

Day 3	Seated Ankle Circles, Seated Hip Circles, Shoulder Rolls | Reverse Kegel, Seated Core Engagement, Basic Kegel | Seated Forward Fold, Pelvic Floor Release	2 sets / 10 reps each	Ch. 4 | Ch. 5 | Ch. 4
Day 4	Seated Knee Lifts, Seated Torso Rotation, Shoulder Rolls | Basic Kegel, Pelvic Tilt, Diaphragmatic Breathing with Movement | Supine Knees to Chest, Pelvic Floor Release	2 sets / 10 reps each	Ch. 4 | Ch. 5 | Ch. 4
Day 5	REST DAY — Light walking encouraged	—	—
Day 6	Seated Ankle Circles, Seated Knee Lifts, Seated Hip Circles | Reverse Kegel, Seated Core Engagement, Basic Kegel | Seated Forward Fold, Pelvic Floor Release	2 sets / 10 reps each	Ch. 4 | Ch. 5 | Ch. 4
Day 7	Full session: All 5 warm-ups | All 5 foundation exercises (1 set each) | All 3 cool-downs	1 set / 8-10 reps each	Ch. 4 + Ch. 5 + Ch. 4

Week 1 Check-In Tracker

Sessions completed (check each day you exercised):

Mon	Tue	Wed	Thu	Fri	Sat	Sun
☐	☐	☐	☐	☐	☐	☐

Which exercise felt most natural this week, and which was hardest to feel?

- -

Did you notice any change in urgency or leakage compared to before starting?

- -

Were there days when finding the pelvic floor muscles felt clearer? What was different?

- -

Energy level this week (circle one):   1   2   3   4   5

Personal win this week:

- -

Week 2 — Activation

Week 2 introduces the core strength exercises from Chapter 6 alongside the foundation work. Sessions become more demanding this week, and that is deliberate. The bridge, clamshell, and supported squat add load to the pelvic floor in a controlled, progressive way that Week 1 has prepared the body for. You may feel more muscular fatigue after sessions than in Week 1. That is appropriate and expected. What should not appear is sharp pain, significant pelvic pressure, or worsening urgency. If any of those occur, reduce the sets of the strength exercises and contact your healthcare provider if they persist beyond 48 hours.

Day	Exercises	Sets / Reps	Chapter Reference
Day 1	Seated Knee Lifts, Seated Torso Rotation, Shoulder Rolls | Basic Kegel (3 sets), Seated Core Engagement, Bridge | Seated Forward Fold, Pelvic Floor Release	2-3 sets / 10 reps	Ch. 4 | Ch. 5 + Ch. 6 | Ch. 4
Day 2	REST DAY	—	—
Day 3	Seated Ankle Circles, Seated Hip Circles, Shoulder Rolls | Reverse Kegel, Clamshell, Supported Squat | Seated Forward Fold, Pelvic Floor Release	2-3 sets / 10-12 reps	Ch. 4 | Ch. 5 + Ch. 6 | Ch. 4
Day 4	Seated Knee Lifts, Seated Torso Rotation, Shoulder Rolls | Basic Kegel (3 sets), Modified Bird-Dog, Standing Side Leg Raise | Supine Knees to Chest, Pelvic Floor Release	2-3 sets / 10 reps	Ch. 4 | Ch. 5 + Ch. 6 | Ch. 4
Day 5	REST DAY	—	—
Day 6	Seated Ankle Circles, Seated Hip Circles, Shoulder Rolls | Reverse Kegel, Wall Sit with Core Activation, Pelvic Tilt | Seated Forward Fold, Pelvic Floor Release	2-3 sets / 10 reps	Ch. 4 | Ch. 5 + Ch. 6 | Ch. 4
Day 7	Full session: All 5 warm-ups | 2 foundation + all 6 strength (2 sets each) | All 3 cool-downs	2 sets / 10 reps each	Ch. 4 + Ch. 5 + Ch. 6 + Ch. 4

Week 2 Check-In Tracker

Sessions completed (check each day you exercised):

Mon	Tue	Wed	Thu	Fri	Sat	Sun
☐	☐	☐	☐	☐	☐	☐

Which strength exercise felt most challenging, and did the difficulty change across the week?

Has your awareness of pelvic floor engagement during movement improved since Week 1?

Are you noticing any changes in urgency, frequency, or confidence in daily activity?

Did you experience soreness after sessions? Where, and did it resolve within 24 hours?

Energy level this week (circle one): 1 2 3 4 5

Personal win this week:

Week 3 — Building

Week 3 is the most demanding week in the program. The bladder control exercises from Chapter 7 are added to every session, and total volume increases across all categories. The Urge Suppression Technique and Bladder Retraining Protocol are integrated into daily life this week, not only during sessions. Most women find that Week 3 is when the clearest functional improvements begin to appear: urge suppression starts to feel like a genuine tool, and the timing of the pelvic floor contraction in daily situations becomes more automatic. Maintain the two rest days. The temptation to push through them is common and counterproductive. Muscle adaptation happens during recovery, not during exercise.

Day	Exercises	Sets / Reps	Chapter Reference
Day 1	Seated Ankle Circles, Seated Knee Lifts, Shoulder Rolls | Basic Kegel, Endurance Holds, Bridge, Clamshell | Quick-Flick Kegels, Functional Kegel (chair rise) | Seated Forward Fold, Pelvic Floor Release	3 sets / 10-12 reps	Ch. 4 | Ch. 5+6 | Ch. 7 | Ch. 4
Day 2	REST DAY — Practice Urge Suppression Technique throughout the day	—	Ch. 7 (daily protocol)
Day 3	Seated Torso Rotation, Seated Hip Circles, Shoulder Rolls | Reverse Kegel, Seated Core Engagement, Supported Squat, Standing Side Leg Raise | Quick-Flick Kegels, Functional Kegel (picking up) | Supine Knees to Chest, Pelvic Floor Release	3 sets / 10-12 reps	Ch. 4 | Ch. 5+6 | Ch. 7 | Ch. 4
Day 4	Seated Ankle Circles, Seated Knee Lifts, Shoulder Rolls | Basic Kegel (3 sets), Endurance Holds, Modified Bird-Dog, Wall Sit | Quick-Flick Kegels, Urge Suppression practice | Seated Forward Fold, Pelvic Floor Release	3 sets / 10-12 reps	Ch. 4 | Ch. 5+6 | Ch. 7 | Ch. 4
Day 5	REST DAY — Continue Bladder Retraining Protocol	—	Ch. 7 (daily protocol)
Day 6	All 5 warm-ups | Reverse Kegel, Pelvic Tilt, Bridge, Clamshell, Supported Squat | Endurance Holds, Functional Kegel (sudden laugh) | All 3 cool-downs	3 sets / 10-12 reps	Ch. 4 | Ch. 5+6+7 | Ch. 4
Day 7	Full session: All warm-ups | 2 foundation + all 6 strength + 3 bladder exercises | All cool-downs	3 sets / 10-12 reps	Ch. 4 + Ch. 5 + Ch. 6 + Ch. 7 + Ch. 4

Week 3 Check-In Tracker

Sessions completed (check each day you exercised):

Mon	Tue	Wed	Thu	Fri	Sat	Sun

☐   ☐   ☐   ☐   ☐   ☐   ☐

Has the Urge Suppression Technique started to feel more effective? Describe one moment when it worked.

____

Which bladder control exercise produced the most noticeable change in your daily symptoms?

____

How has the volume of Week 3 compared to Weeks 1 and 2 in terms of fatigue and recovery?

____

What symptom improvement, however small, are you most grateful for this week?

____

Energy level this week (circle one): 1 2 3 4 5

Personal win this week:

____

Week 4 — Confidence

Week 4 is the consolidation week. The mobility exercises from Chapter 8 are integrated into every session, and the endurance demands of the strength work increase with longer holds and higher set volumes. The focus shifts from learning new exercises to performing all of them with the coordination that four weeks of consistent practice has built. By the end of Week 4, most women can complete a full session of warm-up, foundation, strength, bladder control, and mobility work in under 25 minutes. When Week 4 is complete, repeat it for two more weeks before cycling back to Week 2 to maintain and continue building on the gains this month has produced.

Day	Exercises	Sets / Reps	Chapter Reference
Day 1	All 5 warm-ups	Basic Kegel (3 sets), Bridge (3 sets + 5 single-leg), Clamshell	Quick-Flick Kegels, Functional Kegel	Hip Flexor Stretch, Inner Thigh Release	Pelvic Floor Release	3 sets / 10-12 reps	Ch. 4	Ch. 5+6	Ch. 7	Ch. 8	Ch. 4
Day 2	REST DAY — Bladder Retraining Protocol + Functional Kegel practice throughout day	—	Ch. 7 + Ch. 10
Day 3	All 5 warm-ups	Reverse Kegel, Seated Core Engagement, Supported Squat (3 sets), Standing Side Leg Raise	Endurance Holds (10-sec), Urge Suppression practice	Lower Back Mobility Roll, Cat-Cow with Pelvic Floor Coordination	Pelvic Floor Release	3 sets / 10-12 reps	Ch. 4	Ch. 5+6	Ch. 7	Ch. 8	Ch. 4
Day 4	All 5 warm-ups	Basic Kegel (3 sets), Modified Bird-Dog, Wall Sit (45-sec holds)	Quick-Flick Kegels, Functional Kegel	Seated Figure-Four, Hip Flexor Stretch	Pelvic Floor Release	3 sets / 10-12 reps	Ch. 4	Ch. 5+6	Ch. 7	Ch. 8	Ch. 4
Day 5	REST DAY — Urge Suppression + 10-minute walk focusing on walking posture from Ch. 10	—	Ch. 7 + Ch. 10
Day 6	All 5 warm-ups	Reverse Kegel, Pelvic Tilt, Bridge (3 sets), Clamshell	Endurance Holds, Bladder Retraining check-in	Cat-Cow, Inner Thigh Release	Seated Forward Fold, Pelvic Floor Release	3 sets / 10-12 reps	Ch. 4	Ch. 5+6+7+8	Ch. 4
Day 7	Full program session: All warm-ups	All foundation + all strength + all bladder + all mobility	All cool-downs	3 sets / 10-12 reps	Ch. 4 through Ch. 8 integrated

Week 4 Check-In Tracker

Sessions completed (check each day you exercised):

Mon	Tue	Wed	Thu	Fri	Sat	Sun
☐	☐	☐	☐	☐	☐	☐

How does a full Week 4 session feel compared to your very first Week 1 session?

End-of-Program Self-Assessment

Return to the self-assessment checklist you completed in the Introduction. Read back through your original yes or no answers, then respond to the six reflection questions below. These questions correspond directly to the eight starting-point items. Write your answers honestly. What you have noticed matters more than what you expected to notice.

How to Use This Assessment

This is not a test. There is no passing mark and no expected outcome. Some symptoms improve quickly, others take longer, and some are better addressed with professional support alongside this program. The purpose of these questions is to give you a clear, specific picture of what has changed across four weeks and what direction to take from here.

1. *Has leakage during sneezing, coughing, laughing, or exercise changed? Describe specifically what is different now compared to when you started.*

2. *Has urgency changed? Are you reaching the bathroom more calmly, waiting longer, or using the Urge Suppression Technique successfully? Describe a specific example.*

3. *Has your bathroom frequency during the day or night changed? What is your current typical interval between visits compared to your starting point?*

4. *Has the heaviness or pressure feeling in your pelvic area changed? When do you notice it most now compared to before?*

5. *Has your awareness of your pelvic floor during daily movement changed? Describe a daily moment where you now engage these muscles without consciously thinking about it.*

6. *Has your confidence in physical activity or social situations changed? Is there something you are now doing that you were avoiding or managing around before you started?*

Chapter 10

Life Beyond the Program

The program ends. The habits do not. Everything built across the four weeks, the breathing pattern, the muscle awareness, the urge management, the strength, becomes more stable and more automatic the longer you maintain it. This chapter protects that progress in the hours between sessions.

Foods and Drinks That Affect Your Bladder

The bladder is a muscle, but it is also a mucous-membrane-lined organ that reacts to what passes through it. Certain foods and drinks directly irritate the bladder lining or stimulate the detrusor muscle to contract earlier than it needs to. Understanding which ones affect you does not mean eliminating them permanently. It means making informed choices on days when bladder symptoms are already elevated.

Caffeine is the most significant and consistent bladder irritant. It acts as a diuretic, increasing urine production, and it also directly stimulates the bladder muscle, triggering urgency contractions regardless of how full the bladder actually is. Coffee is the most concentrated source, but tea, cola drinks, energy drinks, and even chocolate contain enough caffeine to affect women with a sensitive bladder. Reducing rather than eliminating is a reasonable starting point: switching from two cups to one, or from caffeinated to decaffeinated in the afternoon, often produces a measurable reduction in urgency within a few days.

Alcohol affects the bladder through two separate pathways. Like caffeine, it increases urine output by suppressing the hormone that signals the kidneys to retain water. It also reduces the brain's inhibitory control over the bladder, so the urge signal arrives with less moderation than usual. Carbonated drinks, including sparkling water, introduce gas pressure into the bladder that can mimic or intensify urgency. Artificial sweeteners, particularly aspartame and saccharin, are known bladder irritants for a subset of women.

Acidic foods and drinks, including citrus fruits, tomato products, and vinegar-based foods, can inflame a sensitive bladder lining and worsen both urgency and frequency.

The hydration paradox is worth addressing directly. Many women with urgency or frequency deliberately reduce how much they drink, reasoning that less fluid means fewer bathroom visits. The opposite is often true. Concentrated urine is significantly more irritating to the bladder lining than diluted urine and can worsen urgency, frequency, and discomfort. Aim for six to eight standard glasses of water across the day, with the larger portion consumed before mid-afternoon to reduce overnight visits.

Common Bladder Irritants and Bladder-Friendly Alternatives

Bladder Irritant	Why It Irritates	Bladder-Friendly Alternative
Coffee and caffeinated tea	Stimulates bladder muscle; increases urine output	Decaffeinated coffee or herbal tea; reduce quantity gradually
Alcohol (all types)	Increases urine output; reduces bladder inhibition	Plain water, herbal tea, or diluted juice
Carbonated drinks	Gas pressure mimics urgency signal	Still water or herbal iced tea
Citrus fruits and juices	Acidifies urine; inflames bladder lining	Pear or apple juice diluted with water
Artificial sweeteners	Direct irritant to bladder lining	Plain water; small amounts of stevia if needed
Tomato products and vinegar	Acidic content inflames bladder lining	Reduce portion; avoid on high-symptom days

Daily Habits That Protect Your Progress

The pelvic floor responds to every load placed on it throughout the day: every time you bend, lift, carry, stand up, walk, or cough. The habits in this section reduce unnecessary load so that the strength you are building in sessions is not being drained by poor mechanics between them.

Safe lifting is the most direct daily application of the skills built in this program. Before lifting anything heavier than a full kettle, exhale first, engage your lower belly lightly, and perform a gentle pelvic floor contraction. Lift as you continue to exhale. This sequence, which the Functional Kegel in Chapter 7 has been training, ensures that core pressure is managed from above and below simultaneously rather than dumped downward onto the pelvic floor as effort begins. Bending from the hips rather than rounding from the lower back also significantly reduces the abdominal pressure generated during the lift.

Getting out of a chair correctly matters given how many times daily this movement occurs. Slide to the front edge of the seat first. Place both feet flat on the floor, hip-width apart. Lean forward from the hips until your shoulders are over your feet, exhale, contract your pelvic floor, and then press through your heels to rise. Avoid pushing up from armrests unless balance requires it, since that technique tends to encourage breath-holding and posterior pelvic tilt, both of which increase downward pressure on the pelvic floor.

Safe Lifting and Chair Rise: Correct Movement Patterns

Walking posture deserves specific attention because walking is the most sustained daily load the pelvic floor manages. A forward head, rounded upper back, or anteriorly tilted pelvis each place the pelvic floor at a mechanical disadvantage with every step. Walk with your weight slightly more toward your heels, your tailbone pointing toward the floor in neutral alignment, and your gaze forward rather than down. This posture activates the gluteus medius, reducing the lateral pelvic drop that otherwise creates repetitive downward pressure on the pelvic floor with every stride.

The discreet daily Kegel habit is one of the most effective ways to maintain pelvic floor function between formal sessions. Link a brief contraction sequence to an existing daily habit so it requires no extra planning. Effective anchor activities include: the first minute of sitting down with tea or coffee in the morning, waiting at a red light, the first two minutes of a television program, standing at the kitchen counter while the kettle boils, and brushing teeth at night. Three to five contractions at each of these anchors adds meaningful training volume without adding a single scheduled session to your day.

Sleep, Stress, and the Pelvic Floor

Stress has a direct and specific effect on pelvic floor function. When the body activates the stress response, cortisol rises and the nervous system shifts into heightened alertness. One of the consistent physical responses to elevated cortisol is increased muscle bracing throughout the torso, including the pelvic floor. Women with already-elevated pelvic floor tension often find their urgency and frequency symptoms are measurably worse during high-stress periods, even when fluid intake and activity levels have not changed. Understanding this connection removes the mystery from the pattern and points toward what helps.

The five-minute evening breathing and release routine below is designed to reverse stress-driven bracing before sleep. Perform it lying on your back on your bed or mat. Begin with three slow diaphragmatic breaths, directing each breath into the belly and lower ribs. On each exhale, consciously release the pelvic floor using the Reverse Kegel technique from Chapter 5. After three breath cycles, move into the Supine Knees to Chest position from Chapter 4 and hold for five slow breaths, allowing the lower back and sacrum to release. Return to flat, extend both legs, and perform five more slow diaphragmatic breath cycles with deliberate pelvic floor release on each inhale. The sequence takes four to six minutes and is among the most consistent tools for reducing overnight urgency in women who carry stress tension into their sleep.

Sleep posture influences the pelvic floor primarily through its effect on the lower back and sacrum. Sleeping on your back with a pillow under your knees is the most neutral position for the pelvic floor and lumbar spine, reducing the anterior pelvic tilt that forward-sleepers often carry. Side sleeping with a pillow between the knees is an effective alternative. Sleeping face-down is the least favorable position: it requires the lumbar spine to maintain extension for hours and creates sustained compression through the anterior pelvic structures.

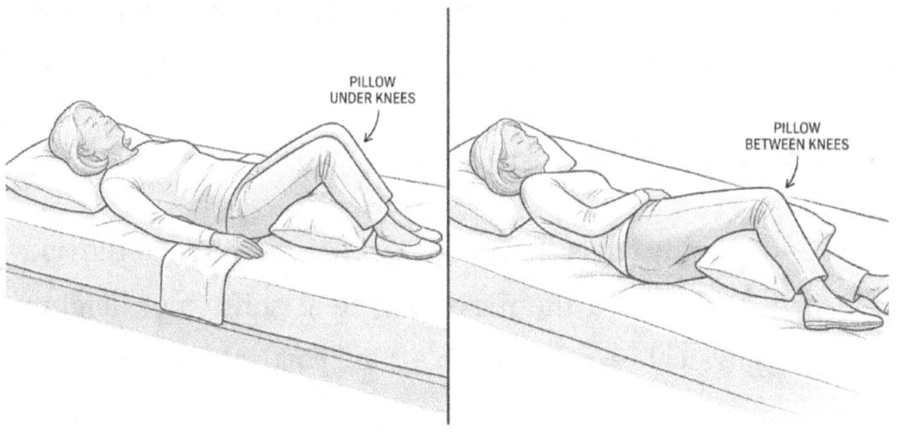

When to Seek More Help

This program addresses a wide range of pelvic floor symptoms safely and effectively. There are specific signs, however, that warrant a conversation with a healthcare provider before or instead of continuing with self-directed exercise alone.

Pain during or after exercise. Discomfort that does not resolve within 24 hours, or that worsens progressively across sessions, requires assessment rather than more exercise.

Significant worsening of symptoms. A marked increase in urgency, frequency, or leakage that develops after beginning the program and does not settle within a week of reduced volume should be discussed with your doctor.

Pelvic pressure or heaviness that increases. A growing sense of heaviness, dragging, or the feeling of something descending into the vaginal area, particularly after standing or exercise, may indicate prolapse that needs professional assessment.

Unexplained bleeding. Any vaginal bleeding after menopause not explained by current hormonal treatment requires prompt medical evaluation.

Inability to empty the bladder or bowel. A new or worsening inability to empty fully, with straining or significant discomfort, should be assessed rather than managed with exercise alone.

Recurring urinary tract infections. More than two UTIs in six months may indicate an underlying structural or hormonal issue that exercise will not resolve.

Numbness or tingling in the pelvic region or inner thighs. Neurological symptoms in the pelvic area warrant medical investigation before any exercise program continues.

No improvement after six to eight consistent weeks. If symptoms have not changed after six to eight weeks of consistent, correct practice, a pelvic floor physical therapist can assess what is limiting progress and provide targeted guidance.

One Conversation Worth Having

A pelvic floor physical therapist is a physical therapist with specialized postgraduate training in the assessment and treatment of pelvic floor dysfunction. An appointment is not a last resort. It is a targeted professional assessment that many women find transforms their self-directed exercise from adequate to highly effective, because the therapist can identify exactly which muscles are underactive, which are overactive, and what specific modifications will produce the fastest results for that individual.

A typical first appointment involves a detailed history of your symptoms, a postural assessment, and, with your consent, an internal examination to assess pelvic floor muscle tone, coordination, strength, and the presence of any trigger points or restricted tissue. The appointment is conducted with complete respect for your comfort and boundaries. You are in control of the pace and extent of the assessment at every point. The therapist will give you a specific diagnosis of your pelvic floor pattern, explain it clearly, and provide a tailored exercise plan that either supplements or replaces what you have been doing.

If you have worked through this full program and want to continue improving, or if your progress has plateaued, or if you simply want professional confirmation of your technique and a personalized next step, asking your primary care physician for a referral to a pelvic floor physical therapist is the single most effective action available to you. It is a conversation worth having.

Did this book give you something?

A stretch you had forgotten. A movement that surprised you. A moment where something clicked and you thought: I can actually feel that.

If it did, a short review on Amazon takes two minutes and costs nothing. For an independent author with no marketing budget, it means everything. It is how the next woman finds this book. It is how someone finds the right gift for a person they care about. It is how this work reaches the hands it was made for.

Search the title on Amazon. One or two honest sentences is all it takes.

Thank you for doing the work. It was a privilege to be part of it.

Conclusion

Four weeks ago you picked up this book for a reason. Maybe it was the leak that caught you off guard, or the urgency that had quietly started dictating where you went and how long you stayed. Whatever brought you here, you stayed. You did the sessions. You learned to breathe differently. You found muscles that most women cannot accurately locate without deliberate guidance. You built a foundation, then built strength on top of it, then applied both to the specific moments in your day that used to feel beyond your control.

That is not a small thing. Most people who buy a health book do not finish it. You did. And the work you completed is not the kind that disappears when the four weeks end. The coordination between your breath, your deep abdominals, and your pelvic floor is now a learned pattern. Learned patterns persist. The Functional Kegel reflex you practiced before chair rises and during sudden laughs has begun to automate. The bladder retraining protocols have interrupted a cycle your bladder had been running on for years. Interrupted cycles do not simply restart on their own.

You now have three specific things you did not have four weeks ago. A stronger core: the diaphragm, transverse abdominis, lower back stabilizers, and pelvic floor working as one coordinated system. Bladder strategies: a practical toolkit you can deploy the moment symptoms appear rather than bracing against them and hoping. And the knowledge to keep going: you understand what your pelvic floor is, how it connects to everything around it, and what to do when things shift.

The next step is straightforward: repeat Week 4 for two more weeks to consolidate the endurance gains, then cycle back to Week 2 and rotate through Weeks 2, 3, and 4 as your maintenance program. Fifteen to twenty minutes a day. That is all it takes to hold and build on what you have established.

I wrote every page of this book with a specific woman in mind: the one sitting across from me in a quiet room, telling me something she had not told anyone else, wondering if anything could actually change. The answer has always been yes. It still is. Go take care of yourself.

Acknowledgements

Writing about the body means listening to people talk about it honestly, which most of us are not raised to do. I am grateful to the women who sat across from me over the years and told me the truth: what hurt, what embarrassed them, what they had given up without telling anyone. Those conversations are the reason every book I write starts where it does, with the real experience, not the clinical version of it.

To the practitioners, physiotherapists, physicians, and researchers whose work quietly underpins everything in these pages: you made it possible to write clearly about things that are genuinely complex. I have tried to do your work justice.

To the women who read early drafts and said "yes, that is exactly it" or "no, that is not how it feels at all": both responses were equally useful. Thank you for the honesty.

And to the reader holding this book: the fact that you picked it up matters. Taking your health seriously is not a small thing, even when it feels like it should be.

About The Author

Calla Holt is a women's movement and wellness educator with more than 15 years of hands-on experience helping women understand and work with their bodies more effectively.

Her career has been built in clinical and community settings, working with women across a wide range of fitness levels, life stages, and starting points. Her focus has always been the same: clear information, honest guidance, and practical programs that work in a real person's real life.

Her background spans pelvic floor rehabilitation, core and postural training, functional movement, bladder health, and the structural changes that shape how women move and feel at every stage of life.

Every book in her series is built on the same foundation: plain-language explanations, exercises tested with real women in real bodies, and a structure that delivers genuine results without requiring a gym, equipment, or hours you do not have.

She writes for women who are done looking for answers that never quite fit.

www.ingramcontent.com/pod-product-compliance
Lightning Source LLC
Chambersburg PA
CBHW080400030726
47598CB00010B/2824